Feel Better Fast

How to Maximize Self-Healing Without Drugs, Injections and Surgery Using the OWL Method™ of Oxygen, Water & Light

By Dr. Chris Cormier, DC

Copyright © 2022 by Dr. Chris Cormier, DC

All Rights Reserved

No part of this publication may be reproduced, distributed, or transmitted in any form or by any means, including photocopying, recording, or other electronic or mechanical methods, or by any information storage and retrieval system without the prior written permission of the publisher, except in the case of very brief quotations embodied in critical reviews and certain other noncommercial uses permitted by copyright law.

Although every effort has been made to ensure the accuracy of the information contained in this book, as of the date of publication, nothing herein should be construed as giving advice. Neither the author nor the publisher assumes responsibility for errors, omissions, or contrary interpretations of the subject matter herein.

The author and publisher do not accept any responsibility for any loss, which may arise as a consequence of reliance on information contained in this book.

ISBN: 978-0-9851333-4-4

Published by The Nerve Health Institute®

Table of Contents

Free Gift for my Readers		iv
Disclaimer		v
Introduction		vi
Chapter 1:	What is the OWL Method™?	1
Chapter 2:	The Power Company	13
Chapter 3:	The Nerve Breaker Box	22
Chapter 4:	The *Hidden Diagnosis* in Elite Athletes	28
Chapter 5:	Why are we OWL Deficient?	34
Chapter 6:	Healing Without DIS (Drugs, Injections, and Surgery)	39
Chapter 7:	What can we do at Home?	46
Chapter 8:	Success Stories with the OWL Method™	52
Conclusion		61
Resources		63
About the Author		66
Other Books by Dr. Chris		67

Free Gift for my Readers

As a way of saying thank you to my readers I have a special gift for you. Use the link below and you'll have instant access to a free gift!

https://www.feelbetterfastathome.com

Disclaimer

Nothing in this book is intended to give individual medical advice or to guarantee results. The success stories described herein are individual and are not promised to be duplicated in all cases. None of the advice herein has been evaluated or approved by the Food and Drug Administration or by any professional medical body or association. I am describing my own professional experiences which I believe to be valid based on my years of practice.

Introduction

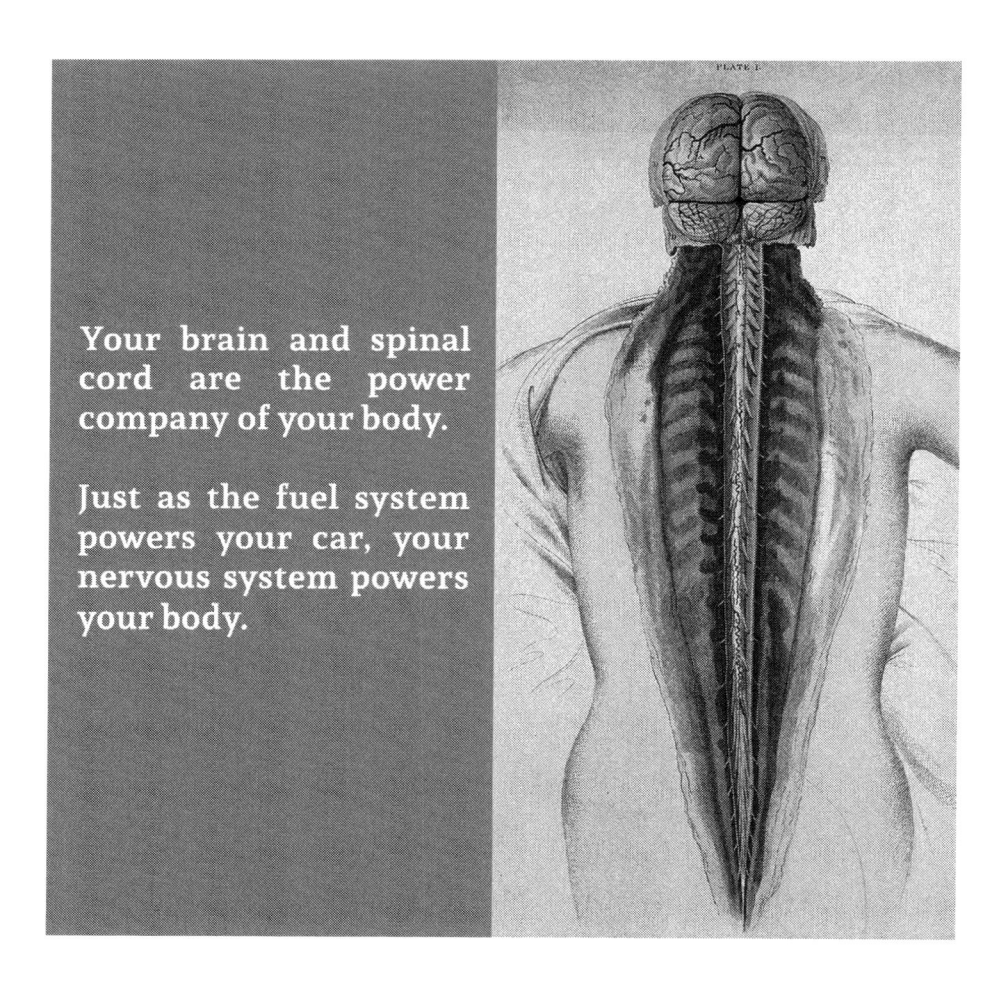

> Your brain and spinal cord are the power company of your body.
>
> Just as the fuel system powers your car, your nervous system powers your body.

I have been a healer for over 20 years. It is my calling to assist our Maker in ensuring that this finely tuned self-healing machine that we have been given is in good working order.

Introduction

You wouldn't drive a car without checking the oil and refilling the gas tank, would you? And you wouldn't fill the gas tank with gasoline tainted with impurities—it would ruin the engine. So why would you run this beautiful body of yours without checking on its essential system—the nervous system—and making sure it has everything it needs to be in good working order?

Your brain and spinal cord are the power company of your body. Just as the fuel system powers your car, your nervous system powers your body. I've learned from experience that about half the health of your power system comes from your parents—that's genetics—and half comes from regular maintenance and health. Some of us are born driving a Ferrari and some of us are born driving a Yugo.

These thoughts are what have driven me in my practice to find the most effective ways to help people feel better faster without drugs, injections, or surgeries. This is how I discovered the OWL Method™. The OWL Method™ is a system of routine maintenance for our bodies that can help keep us in tip-top working order. Oxygen, Water, and Light are the human body's top 3 ingredients needed to sustain quality of life. Deficiencies in these key ingredients lead to decline in good health. On the contrary, adding these 3 important "fuels" to our bodies, and maintaining them, can greatly improve overall health and wellness.

Our gas and oil—oxygen, water, and light—have been artificially depressed in modern times. We live in a world of processed foods and corn syrup-laden beverages and fluorescent lights. In a perfect world, we would have a "check engine" light come on in our bodies when we have something wrong. We could then head to a mechanic who could run a system check and we would be able to fix our health problems right away by replacing a part or adding new oil. But the human body is way more complex than a car. We do have systems in place to alert us of problems in

vii

our bodies. Aches, pain, numbness, tingling, burning, throbbing, fever, illnesses, etc. are just a few of our "check engine" lights. Many of us ignore these warnings and try quick fixes to just get through the day. These quick fixes can be anything from NSAIDs (Non-Steroidal Anti-Inflammatory Drugs), OTC (over-the-counter) medications, injections, and even surgeries. These methods are oftentimes just addressing the symptom and not the cause. I truly believe that the OWL Method™ can help get to the root of any ailment and our amazing machine (the body) can heal itself better than any outside influence can.

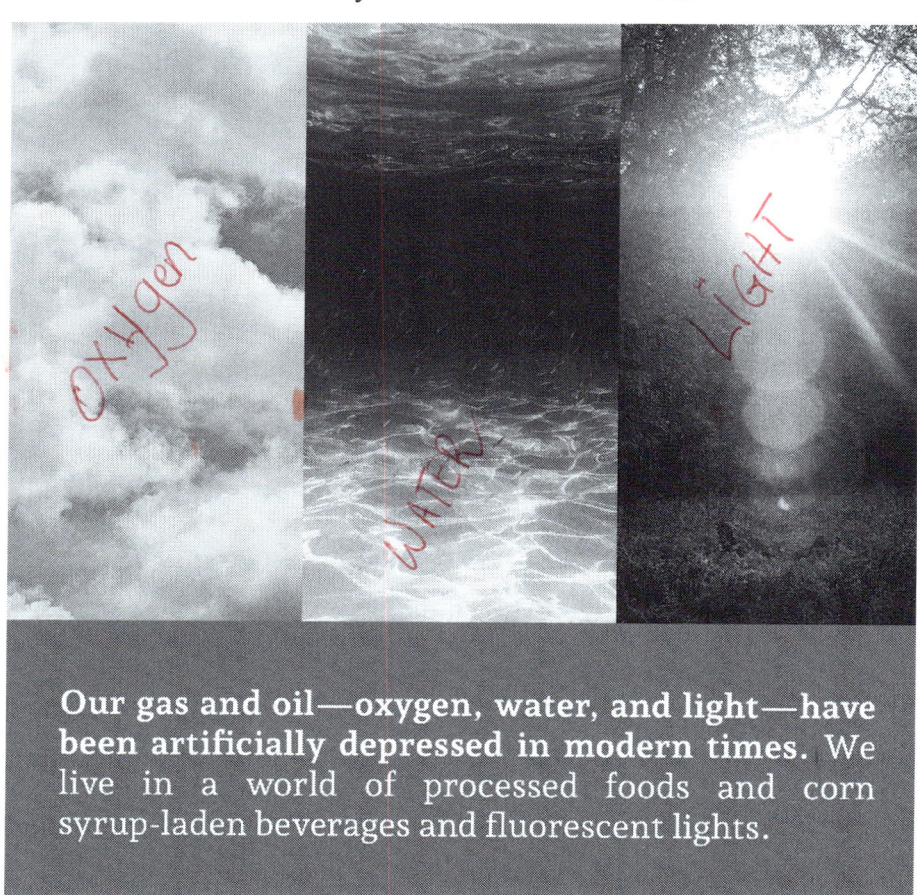

Our gas and oil—oxygen, water, and light—have been artificially depressed in modern times. We live in a world of processed foods and corn syrup-laden beverages and fluorescent lights.

Introduction

The purpose of this book is to teach you how your body really works and how you can help yourself achieve optimum health at any age. Overall, the goal is to help you be healthy. Whether you are driving a Ferrari or a Yugo, you need to maintain your "vehicle" with proper care and maintenance. Just as it is possible to drive a well-maintained car for hundreds of thousands of miles, it is also possible to have a high quality of life for many years.

> **Whether you are driving a Ferrari or a Yugo, you need to maintain your "vehicle" with proper care and maintenance.** Just as it is possible to drive a well-maintained car for hundreds of thousands of miles, it is also possible to have a high quality of life for many years.

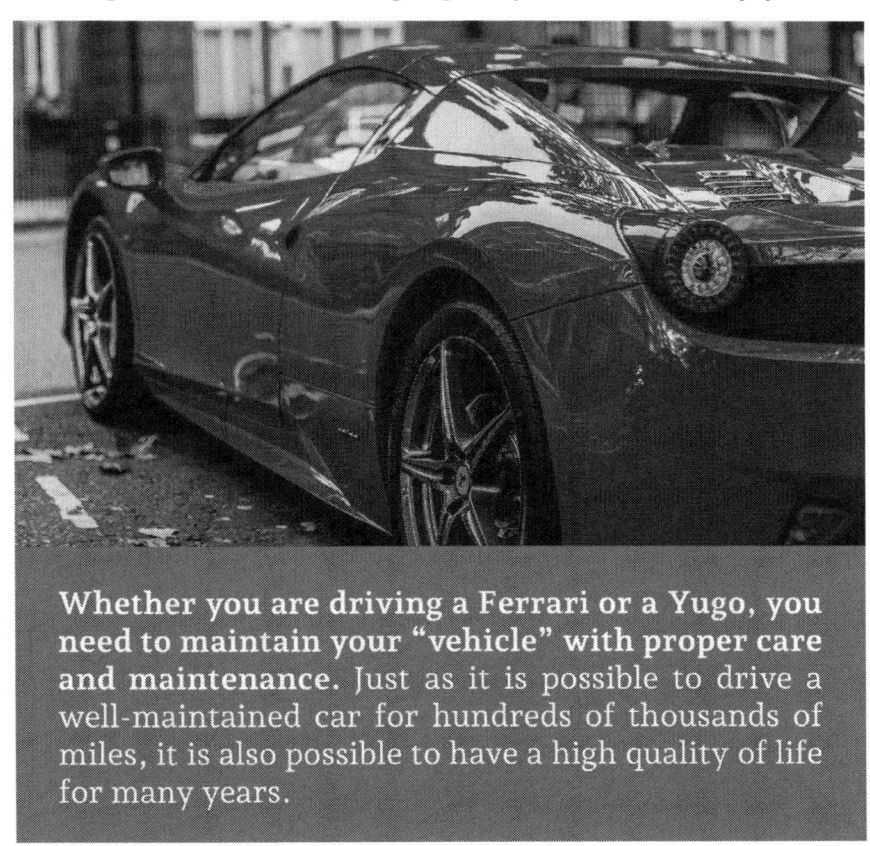

I have used this OWL Method™ on myself as well as on my family and patients. A few years ago, my home was undergoing a renovation and we were moving some furniture in my dining room. Not realizing how low the light fixture was when we moved the dining room table out, I hit the top of my head very hard on the metal base of the chandelier. I immediately fell to

ix

the ground and saw stars. By the next morning, I had paralysis in my right arm (my dominant arm) and severe right neck and upper back pain. I could not treat patients and I could not drive. I also had trouble with simple tasks like eating and putting in my contact lenses. I went from being completely normal to barely able to function and that was very frightening. I went to get a cervical MRI and the diagnosis was a concussion and cervical radiculopathy. The suggested treatment was immediate surgery to alleviate the pressure on the spinal cord and nerves. A second opinion involved no surgery but offered rest with physical therapy and injections. My life's work prepared me for this exact moment. It was the worst injury I had ever had and a very scary thought to be down and out. I realized that I could self-heal more quickly if I put in the work and got to the root cause of my problem. An injury that big cannot have a quick fix. The wrong course of treatment can change the direction of your health forever.

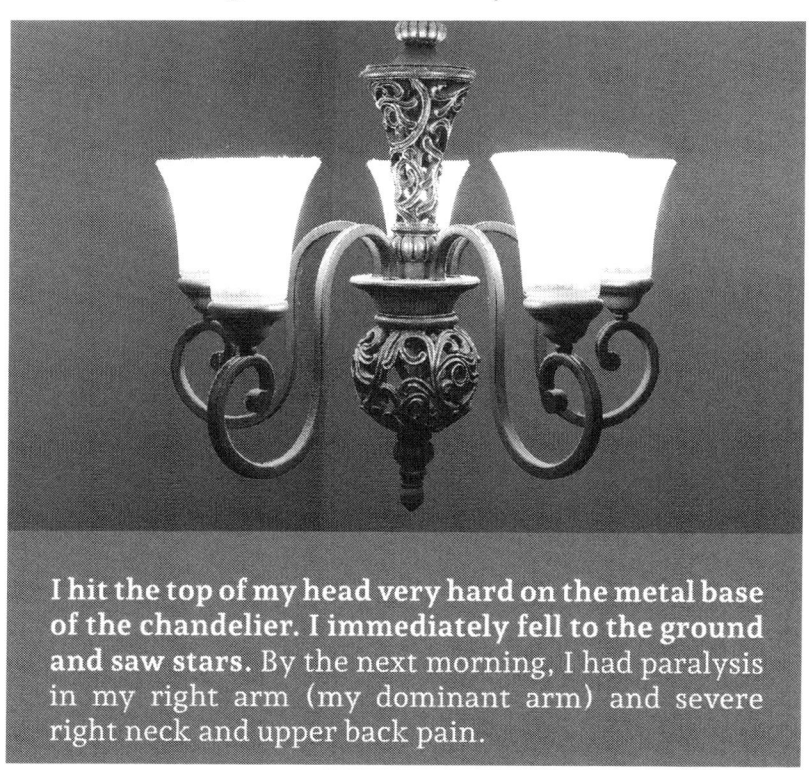

> **I hit the top of my head very hard on the metal base of the chandelier. I immediately fell to the ground and saw stars.** By the next morning, I had paralysis in my right arm (my dominant arm) and severe right neck and upper back pain.

Introduction

I immediately sought the advice of my colleague, Dr. Ed Chauvin. He is a fellow chiropractic physician who practices the advanced technique of Quantum Neurology®, which uses nerve testing and light therapy to rehabilitate nerve weaknesses. Throughout my healing process, the birth of the OWL Method™ began. I had been using hydration, Quantum Neurology®, and light in my practice for years but oxygen and advanced light devices were not as prevalent.

Within 6 weeks of my original injury, and without the use of drugs, injections, or surgery, I was 85–90 percent better. I resumed almost all of my former activities and was on the road to complete recovery. This injury led to the discovery of the importance of oxygen and advanced light therapy in healing the body and so I added these advancements to my practice. I also improved upon the water and light treatments that I had been using for years.

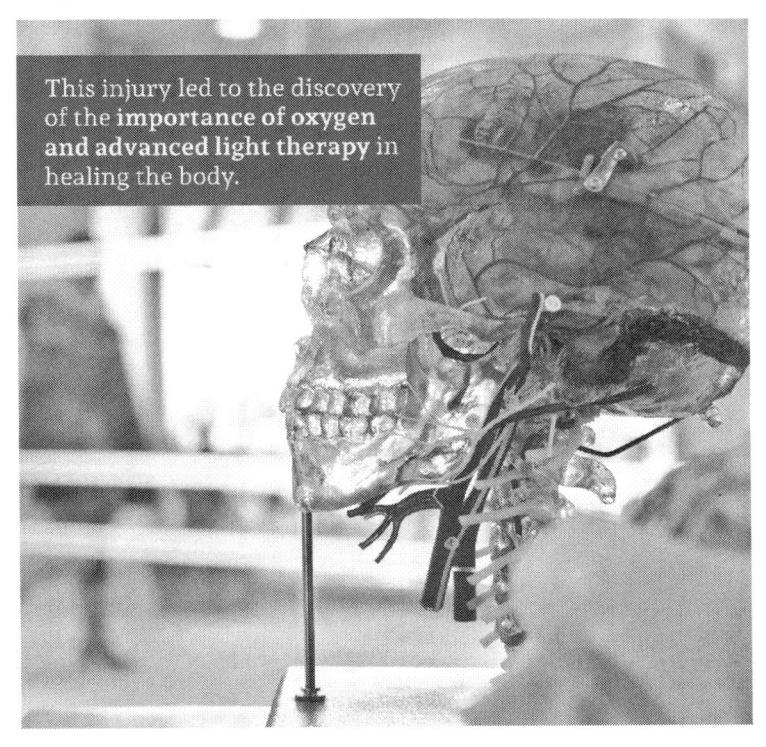

> This injury led to the discovery of the **importance of oxygen and advanced light therapy** in healing the body.

I am my own success story! I truly believe God brought me to this point so that I am better able to serve my patients. I understood, through my own experience, that getting to the root cause of the problem was always going to be better in the end. Using oxygen, water, and light saved my health and it can save yours too!

We have an office filled with devices and methods unlike any other clinic. I'd love to have each and every one of you as a patient and see you walk into my office and walk out feeling better and self-healing better. I understand that not all of you have the resources to travel to see me. Time and money, travel and distance are all factors.

That's why at the end of this book, you'll find a resource section. Whenever I talk about what you should be doing or putting into your body, or a particular type of treatment that might help you, check the resources section to see how you can find that nutritional supplement, treatment, or the brands I like best.

Let's get to FEELING BETTER FAST!

Chapter 1

What is the OWL Method™?

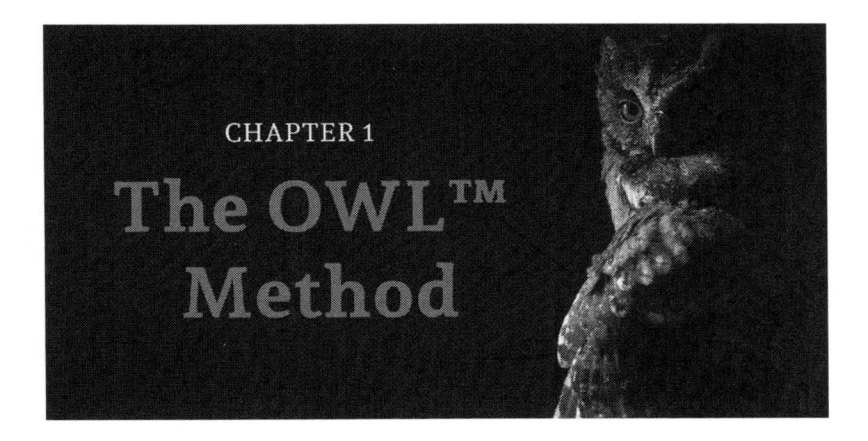

Conventional healthcare methodology has a few tools in its box: medicines, injections, and surgeries. Sometimes these tools work. Sometimes these tools are very necessary. But more often than not, these tools are overused and even abused.

I'm going to show you a new box with new tools in it that may very well allow you to fix what's broken in an innovative way without those drastic measures. That new box contains the OWL Method™. The OWL Method™ is based on the idea that your cells primarily need 3 essential ingredients to be healthy and fully functioning: Oxygen, Water, and Light.

Your body is made up of trillions of cells. Each cell needs a significant amount of oxygen, water, and light to be healthy. Let's take each of these in turn and see in detail how they keep our bodies working.

Oxygen

Our most vital function is breathing and most of us are aware that this is because of the need for oxygen from the air. There is less of it than we might think—most air has only 21 percent oxygen. The rest is made up of other gases such as nitrogen, argon, helium, carbon dioxide, and things like water vapor. There are also many pollutants, toxins, and chemicals in air, which is why, now more than ever, oxygen is most important for overall health and wellness.

We need oxygen to live. Our red blood cells are only red because of the oxygen in our bloodstream. They absorb oxygen in our lungs and take it around our body to feed our cells. By the time the red blood cells get back to the lungs to refresh their oxygen supplies, they are a purplish/bluish color. Oxygen is what makes us blush and gives our lips and nailbeds a healthy color. It's not just a metaphor when people say, "You're turning blue." That's a severe case of a lack of oxygen.

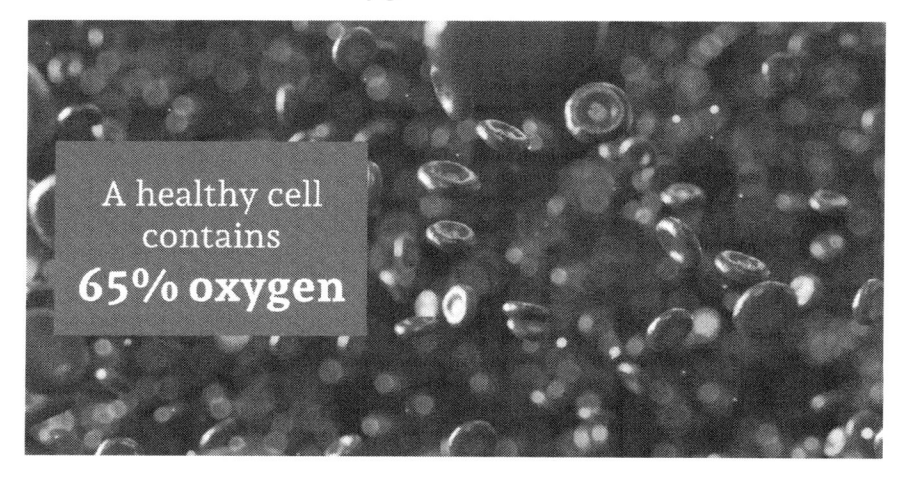

A healthy cell contains **65% oxygen**

A healthy cell contains 65 percent oxygen. In today's methods, oxygen is measured by using a pulse oximeter. This device clamps onto your thumb or finger, and gives a digital percentage of oxygen detected in the blood. Unfortunately, there is not any current device that measures oxygen concentration in each of our trillions of cells at any given moment.

We believe that in today's world everyone is oxygen deficient and consequently, everyone should be doing something to periodically maintain and replenish oxygen.

Methods for re-introducing oxygen into the cells

There are a number of methods for re-introducing oxygen into the cells when someone is operating with an oxygen deficit.

A very simple method to get more oxygen is to BREATHE MORE! We don't breathe enough and oftentimes we shallow breathe. A simple suggestion to help is, every hour, take a few deep breaths in and out.

We're all familiar with the picture of someone strapped to an oxygen tank with a cannula in their nose shooting pure oxygen directly into their airstream. However, this is a pretty radical and inconvenient solution.

In my office, I offer methods that either push oxygen into cells or create a demand for it.

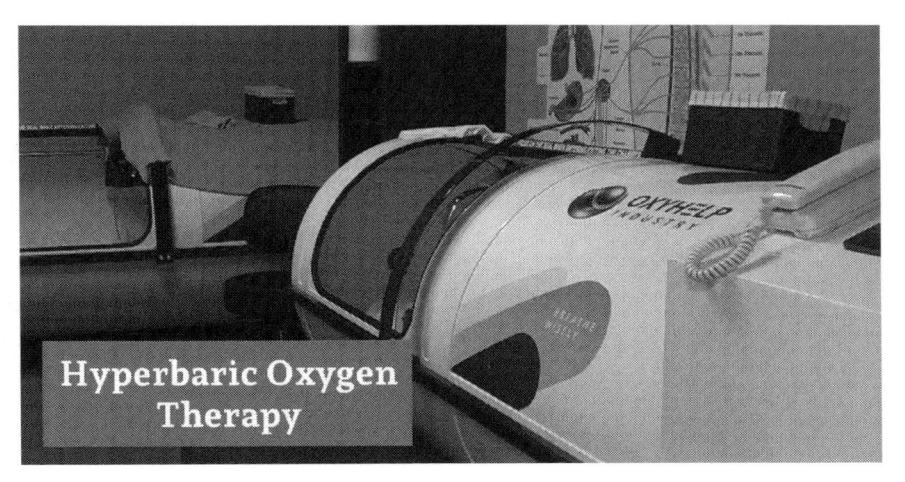

Hyperbaric Oxygen Therapy

Hyperbaric Oxygen Therapy, also known as HBOT, is a method that we offer which pushes oxygen into your cells through pressure. With HBOT, you spend short periods of time in a pressurized chamber while breathing in 94 percent oxygen. This technology was originally developed to treat "the bends" in deep sea divers, but it has been found to be extremely useful in treating oxygen deficits in a variety of situations. It softens the brain-to-blood barrier and makes your cells more readily able to accept this intense flow of pressurized oxygen.

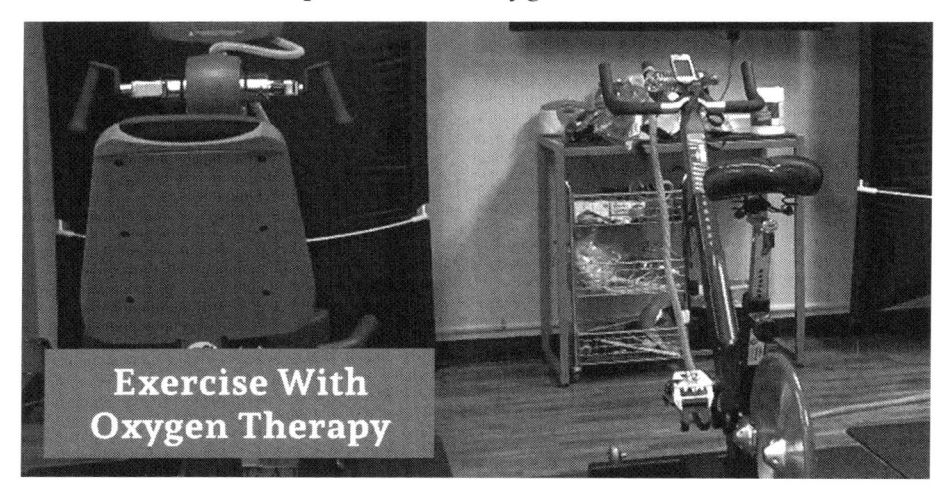

Another method we use is called Exercise with Oxygen Therapy (EWOT). Our patients breathe 94 percent oxygen with their private, sealed masks while exercising for up to 15-minute intervals. This creates a demand for oxygen in all cells involved in exercise and instead of breathing 21 percent oxygen, patients breathe in 94 percent.

When your cells are properly oxygenated, you may find that any inflammation in your bones and the adjacent tissues is reduced. It may also help regenerate blood vessels and other tissues that have had a sluggish regrowth.

You know how you feel when you push yourself running or exercising—how tired you feel, and how you are sucking wind. That's how your cells feel when they don't have enough oxygen. They don't have the energy they need to function properly. They can't do what your body needs them to do. HBOT and EWOT are a quick injection of life into these cells, and once they have more of your body's top ingredient, it's so much easier to maintain higher level body functioning and quality of life.

We make use of HBOT or EWOT in my office, but not everyone lives in Louisiana or is willing or able to make the trip to see me. Check the resources section to see how you might be able to find HBOT or EWOT in your area.

Water

Your body should be more than half water—over 65 percent salt water to be precise. The most efficient method for obtaining water into our cells is by drinking it and absorbing it through our digestive tract. We can also absorb water through our skin just as we can lose water through our sweat and other bodily secretions. We generally recommend drinking half of your body weight (lbs) in ounces per day to achieve proper cellular hydration.

Most of us are used to that sluggish feeling that dehydration brings on. It feels "normal" to us, so we don't think anything of it. Many common ailments can be easily eradicated by simply drinking more water and making sure you are properly hydrated each day.

Methods for re-introducing water into the cells

The simplest and best method for re-introducing water into your cells is by drinking water. This isn't the same thing as drinking liquids, you have to drink *water*.

> The simplest and best method for re-introducing water into your cells is by **drinking water.**

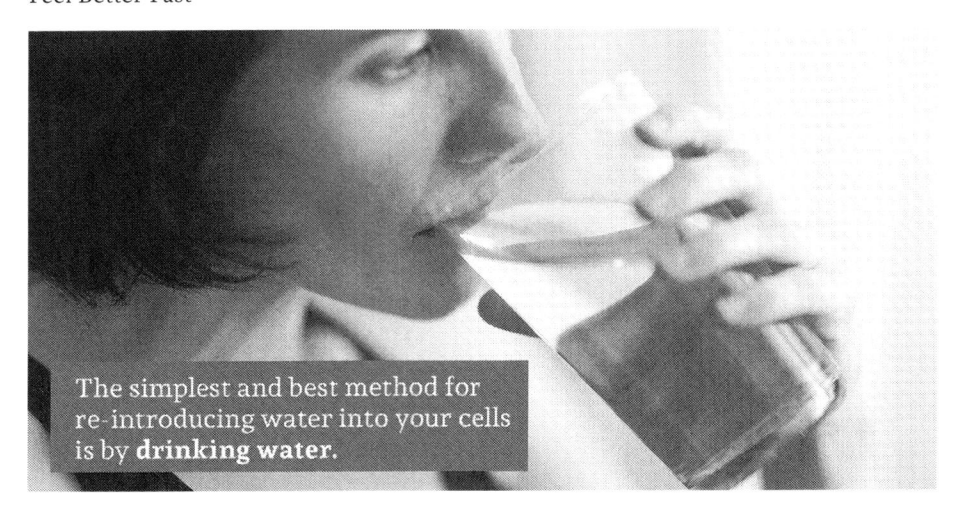

Many people start their day with a cup of coffee or two. There's nothing wrong with that. Coffee tastes good, and when done right it is an organic, natural stimulant. However, caffeine in coffee, cola, teas, etc. dehydrates your cells so the water in your coffee/cola/teas is lost. The same holds true with alcoholic beverages. The body needs to rehydrate after ingesting these other liquids. If you maintain a healthy balance and stay properly hydrated, you can improve your daily quality of life.

Americans also tend to be addicted to processed and refined salt. The average American eats 3.4 grams of processed salt a day, which is far more than the 1.5 grams recommended by the World Health Organization. Aside from the effect refined salt can have on raising your blood pressure and other health issues, salt draws the moisture from your cells into places you don't want it to be. That's why you feel bloated or your feet might swell after you've had a plate of delicious, salty fries. There are better options for salt that are not processed or refined. (Please see the resources section at the end of the book for my salt recommendations.)

Salt is necessary, but water is more necessary. You need water to counterbalance all that salt.

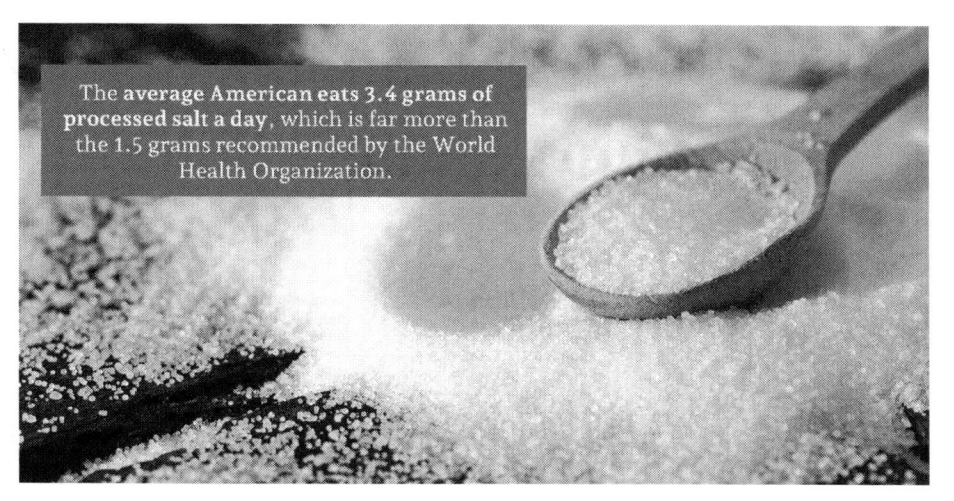

> The **average American eats 3.4 grams of processed salt a day**, which is far more than the 1.5 grams recommended by the World Health Organization.

The recommended amount of water you should consume is half of your body weight in ounces. For instance, a 105-pound woman should be drinking 52.5 ounces of water a day, whereas a 250-pound man should be drinking 125 ounces of water per day.

You also need to consider what kind of water you are putting into your body. Not all water is the same. We live in a world full of pesticides and other pollutants that contaminate the groundwater in many places. Old lead pipes leach into the plumbing systems in some areas. There are also bad ingredients in water bottles. You want to make sure that your water is as pure as possible. The last thing you want to do is rehydrate with toxins.

See the resources section for my recommendations for water and filtration systems.

Light

When we think of light, we think of the visible spectrum of light. A beam of light actually contains the colors of the rainbow—red, orange, yellow, green, blue, indigo, and violet. We get light from the sun, as well as from fire, light bulbs and from the glow of our electronic devices. These forms of light are all visible.

Light is so much more than just what we can see. The true definition of light includes the entire electromagnetic spectrum, most of which humans can't see or even perceive. These forms of invisible light are microwaves, radio waves, infrared rays, ultraviolet rays, and zero-point energy.

While it is easy to understand the effects of oxygen and water on our bodies, and it is easy to understand how to introduce oxygen and water back into our bodies when there is a deficiency, the concept of light being a primary ingredient in the human body is a bit more difficult to understand.

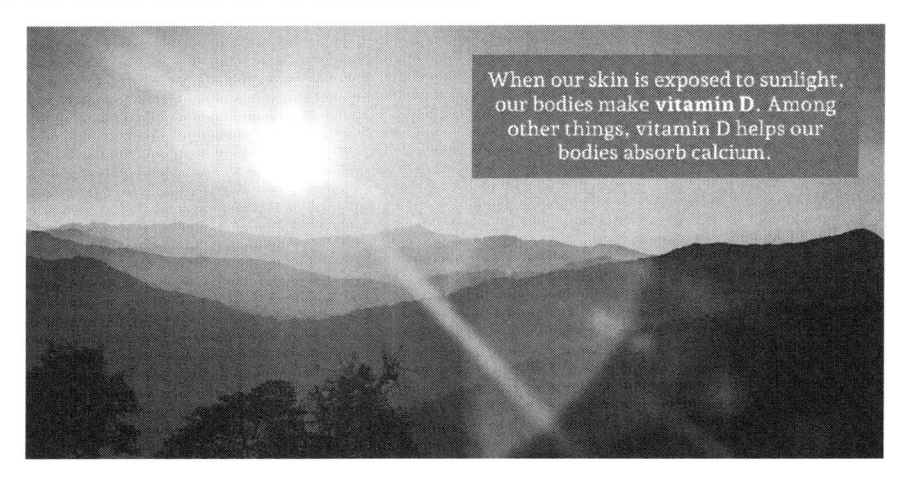

When our skin is exposed to sunlight, our bodies make **vitamin D**. Among other things, vitamin D helps our bodies absorb calcium.

When our skin is exposed to sunlight, our bodies make vitamin D. Among other things, vitamin D helps our bodies absorb calcium. If we don't have enough vitamin D, our bodies suffer. It primarily affects our bones and can lead to osteoporosis and fractures. In rare cases, children with vitamin D deficiency can get rickets, which causes bones to become soft and bend.

Often, you won't experience any symptoms of vitamin D deficiency until it is a serious condition. When symptoms do occur, they are likely to be back or joint pain, weakness, fatigue, or mood changes. You might experience nausea and vomiting as well or become constipated and experience weight problems. There's even an association between a vitamin D deficiency and schizophrenia. It is usually diagnosed by way of a blood test.

These are known problems with light in the human body, but there is a much larger problem lurking in human beings. There is a "Hidden Diagnosis" (the title of my first book) that everyone has and no one knows about.

Your brain and spinal cord are your body's power company. This is where the majority of your body's power (light electricity) is stored. There are 44 pairs of nerves that come off the spinal cord. These nerves start as larger branches but then turn into microscopic branches. Imagine that every millimeter of every organ, bone, skin or muscle in your body is wired by a nerve that connects to your brain and spinal cord!

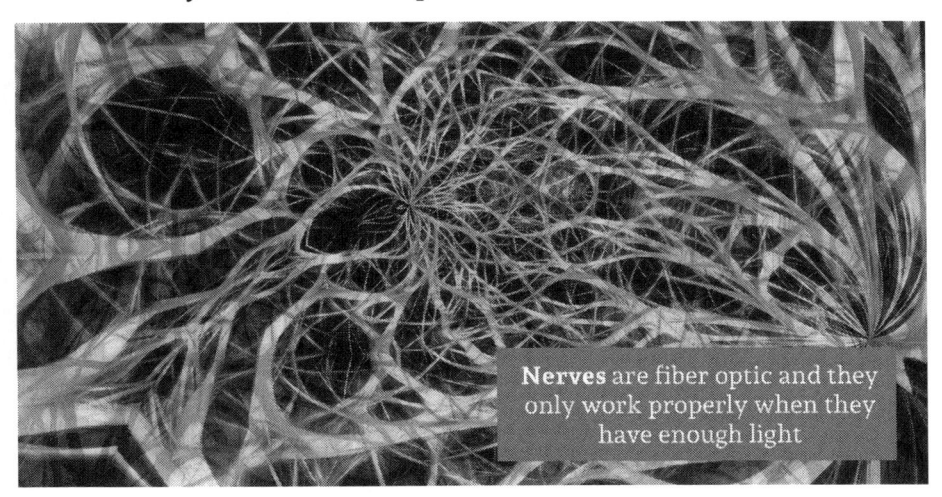

Nerves are fiber optic and they only work properly when they have enough light

Nerves are fiber optic and they only work properly when they have enough light. In other words, it's taking a certain amount of light right now to power my muscles and bones to type these words. Light is not only needed for output like powering and moving muscles and bones, it is also needed for input, like feeling each letter on my keypad.

It is incredibly fascinating when you think of how we were designed and engineered.

There is not a single human being on planet Earth right now who has every millimeter of every nerve connected 100 percent with light. Everyone has power or light outages which are the hidden diagnosis! It is in your best interest to seek out ways to check and restore light in your nervous system to maximize your health. Please check the resources section to see how you might be able to find ways to check and restore your body's light.

Methods for re-introducing light into the cells

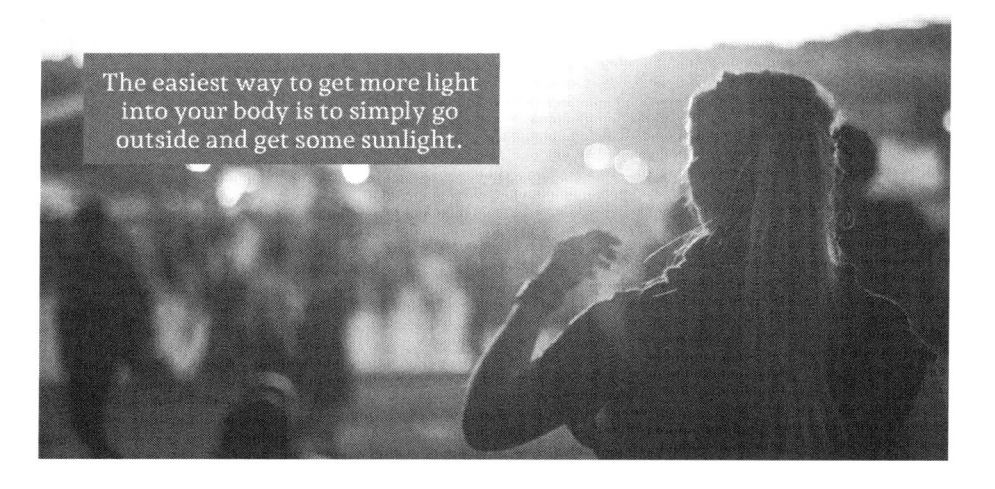

> The easiest way to get more light into your body is to simply go outside and get some sunlight.

The easiest way to get more light into your body is to simply go outside and get some sunlight. Of course, this isn't always an option as climates vary and weather can be a factor. Work schedules and the time of year can prohibit your access to sunshine. Full spectrum lamps designed to mimic sunlight can sometimes help with this.

What is the OWL Method™?

People with Seasonal Affective Disorder, which is a mood disorder brought on by the lack of sunlight in the winter months when the days are short, can greatly benefit from full spectrum lamps as well. Bear in mind that these lamps are *not* the same as tanning lamps or tanning beds. Those are different types of light (ultraviolet) that go out of their way to increase melanin production in your skin and may actually damage it. Be sure to check out our resources section regarding my recommendations for light devices for home use.

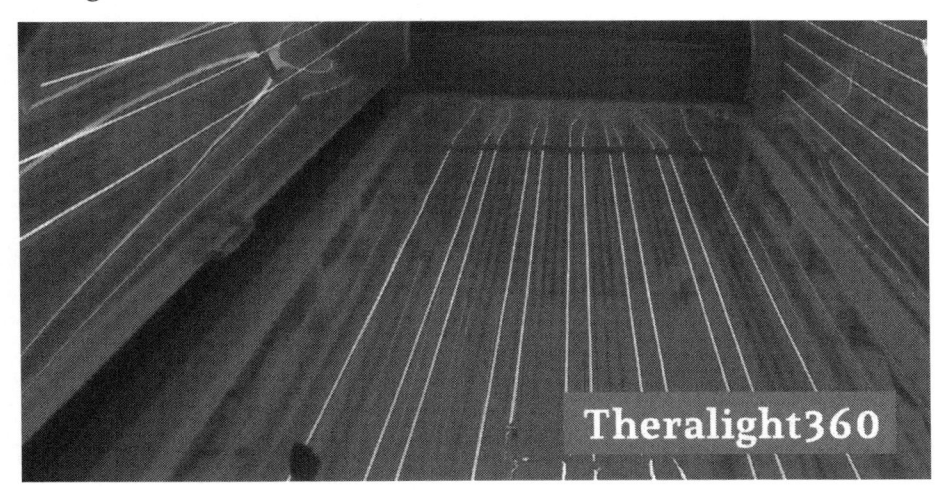

Theralight360

To help get light to every cell in the body, we have in my office one of the most powerful light beds invented. It has 45,000 red and infrared lights and looks like a tanning bed, but without ultraviolet light. It's called a Theralight360, and patients lie in it, unclothed, in a private room, to get maximum absorption into all cells.

We also make use of Contour Light®. Contour Light® has particular frequencies of red and infrared light that is FDA-approved for fat reduction, pain reduction and inflammation reduction. Everyone's body reacts differently to light, but usually after even just one session, you see a difference. With a good diet, we see patients lose many pounds of fat. This light also recharges cells in the body and makes our patients feel really relaxed, and also helps with pain and inflammation.

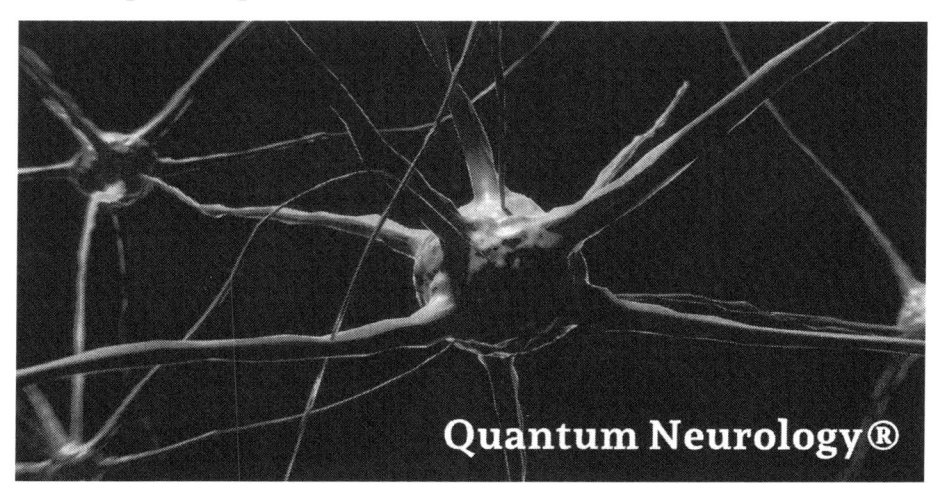

Quantum Neurology®

In order to specifically find and restore light power outages in the body, Advanced Quantum Neurology® is the method we recommend. Similar to a black belt in karate, it takes a trained doctor years to master this technique. Quantum Neurology® was discovered by Dr. George Gonzalez in order to help his 28-year-old wife heal from a supposed permanent condition called cauda equina syndrome whereby she was wheelchair-bound. She has been 100 percent better for more than 15 years now. Quantum Neurology® uses a method of checking and restoring power to weakened nerves. I started my training with Dr. Gonzalez in 2008, and since then I've been so blessed to have witnessed many miracles with my patients, family and friends. It truly has been one of the best things I could have mastered to help someone immediately. If it's not torn or broken, we are oftentimes able to see immediate results. To see my recommendations for full spectrum lights and how to find a Quantum Neurologist® near you, see the resources section at the end of this book.

Chapter 2

The Power Company

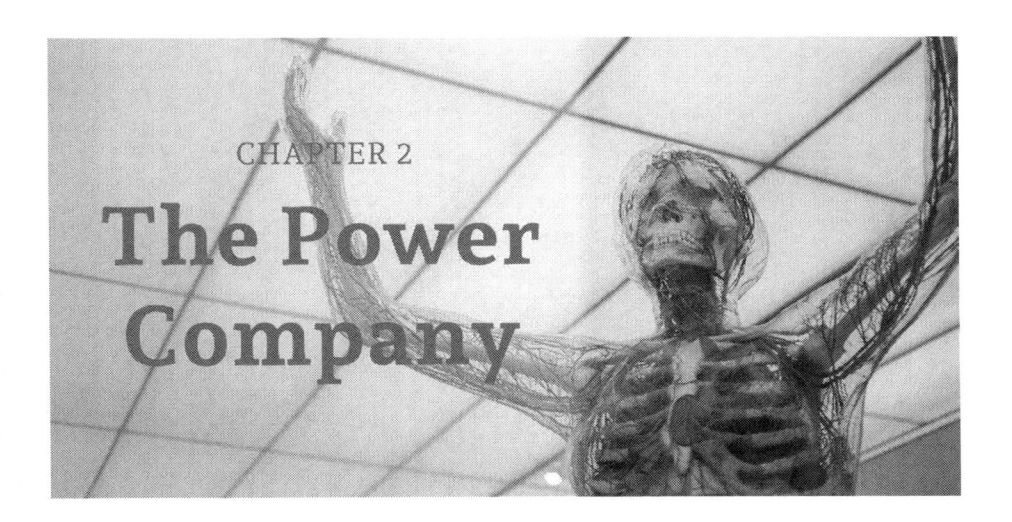

Your nervous system powers your body. Your brain is the powerhouse that sends messages to the rest of your body. Those messages tell your body what to do. Without a correct reading of those messages, there will be malfunctions.

Imagine your nervous system is like a tree and your spinal cord is the trunk. There are 44 main branches of nerves coming off the main trunk, or 88 in total—one set of 44 for your left side and one set of 44 for your right side. Each of these 88 nerves has smaller nerves that branch off them to reach every part of your body.

These nerves give signals that tell your body what to do. They tell your eyelids to blink, your heart to beat, and your legs to move when you walk. They interpret the light that comes in through your eyes and give you sight. They translate the sound waves that enter your ears into what you hear. Everything you sense is transmitted by a nerve impulse into your brain. Every twitch of every muscle fiber, whether voluntary or involuntary, occurs because a nerve communicated it to do so.

Brain and Spinal Cord

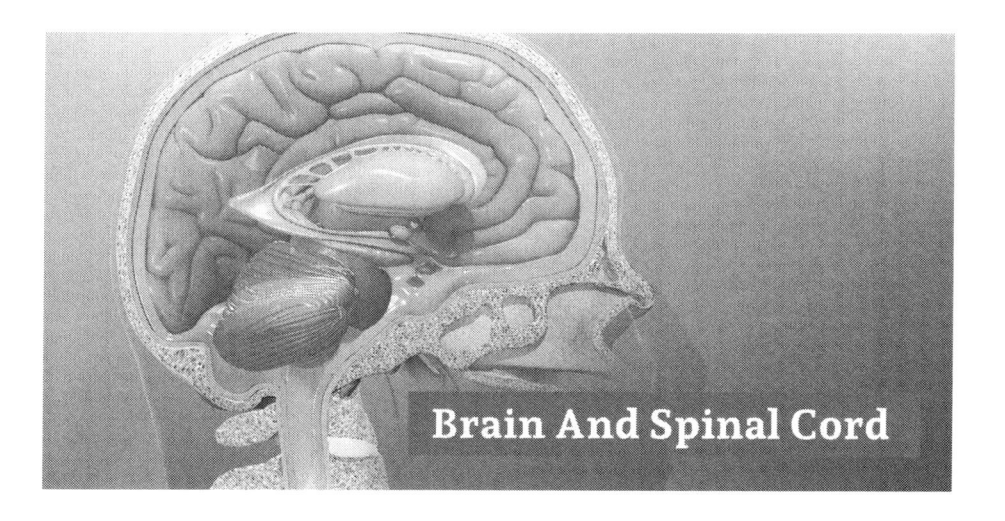

In order for this amazing nervous system to work, there has to be good communication between the brain and the spinal cord. If the message gets garbled between the brain and the spinal cord, there's no chance it will make it intact all the way to its intended recipient.

Remember playing the game of telephone as a kid? You would whisper something into the ear of the person next to you, and they'd whisper it into the ear of the person next to them, and so on down the line. It was always fun to see how tangled the original message got by the time the last person received the message. That game produced a lot of laughs, but it isn't funny if the same thing happens in the communication chain of nerves in your body.

If your stove is on and your hand touches the heating element, you should feel it within milliseconds and pull your hand away to avoid serious injury. Your brain and the nerves in your hand work together to say, "It's hot! Move your hand!" The message travels so quickly from the various nerves in your hand into the brain and the spinal cord that you don't even realize the level of communication taking place. If the nerves in your hand aren't working at full capacity, or if there is some interruption in the spinal cord on the way down to the hand, then your hand might not "get the message" fast enough and a bad burn can occur.

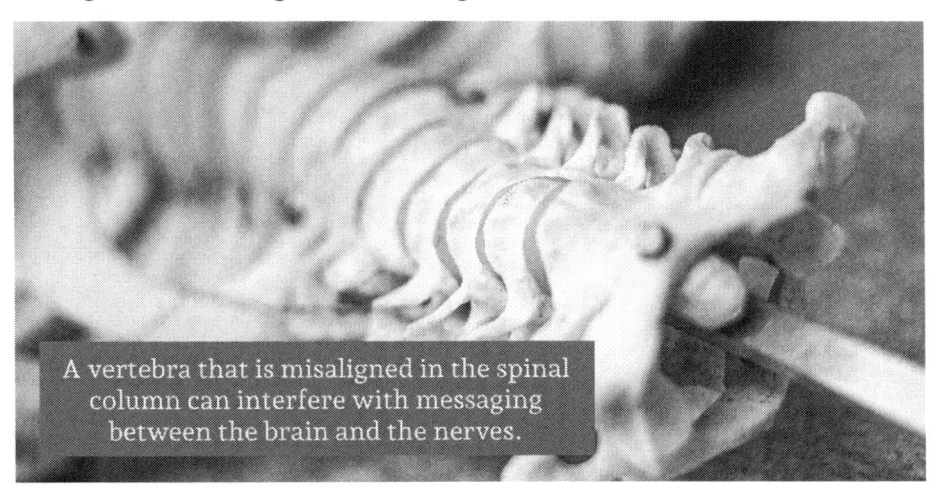

A vertebra that is misaligned in the spinal column can interfere with messaging between the brain and the nerves.

As chiropractic physicians, we make spinal adjustments to alleviate pressure on the spinal nerves. A vertebra that is misaligned in the spinal column can interfere with messaging between the brain and the nerves. There should not be anything that gets in the way of the connection between the brain and spinal cord and all the nerves. Just like it's hard to hear when you have a bad connection on the telephone, you don't want your nerves to have a bad connection when they're receiving signals.

This is what I learned in chiropractic school over 20 years ago. There have been many advancements in the theories of chiropractic and I have adopted what I believe to be the best new treatment protocols to help the body heal without drugs, injections, or surgeries. I have found that the most effective treatment protocols include a combination of the knowledge from the basic principles I learned in undergraduate, doctorate, and post-doctorate schools, in addition to the years of practical knowledge of trying to figure out how to resolve my patients' health conditions. Quantum Neurology® has been one of the best techniques I have mastered to be able to help my patients, family, and friends. It is a method of assessing and instantaneously restoring power to weak nerves in the body.

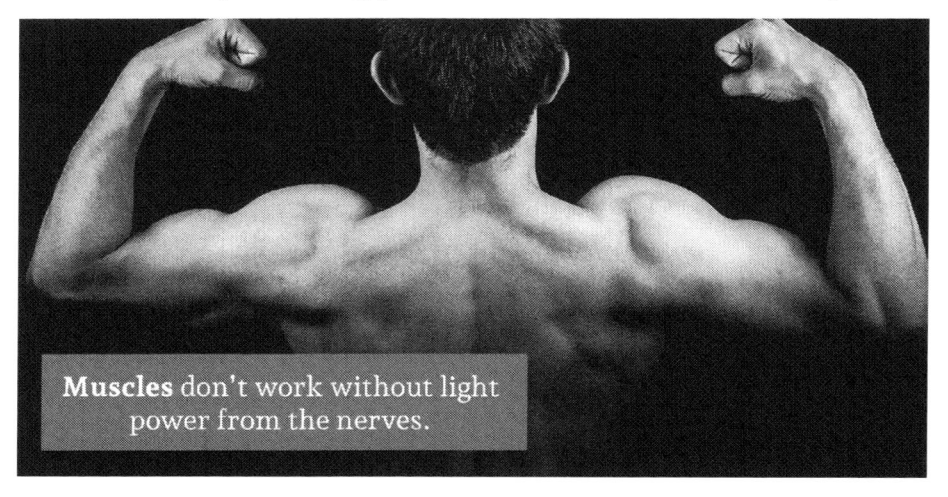

Muscles don't work without light power from the nerves.

The power running through nerves is LIGHT. In other words, moving your finger requires your brain and spinal cord to send light down through nerves to give power to the muscles. Muscles don't work without light power from the nerves. Technically, nerves are fiber optic and this makes the use of light extremely effective in their rehabilitation. In order to test a nerve for a weakness, one must know how it is connected to or from the brain and spinal cord. Quantum Neurology® is an amazing method for assessing the light power in nerves in the body. There are specific techniques from Quantum Neurology® that test weaker nerves by comparing them to stronger ones. Once a QN practitioner finds a weak nerve, they can take the steps needed to rehabilitate that weakness. This often gets rid of symptoms immediately.

88 nerves

Right now, scientists are aware of 44 pairs of major nerves coming off the spinal cord. Our bodies are more or less symmetrical, so we have one for each side of our body which makes for 88 nerves. These nerves branch microscopically and 3 dimensionally into every millimeter of your body.

Nerves need light to work properly!

Most people are familiar with nerves losing function due to being pinched. This can certainly cause interference and loss of light power in the nerve's distributing branches. What most people don't know is that nerves DON'T HAVE TO BE PINCHED to lose power.

At any given moment, nerves can lose light power to parts of your body due to a variety of reasons:

1. Physical stress
2. Emotional stress
3. Biochemical stress

These stresses can cause momentary interference or "short circuits" in nerves. Sometimes the body automatically reboots these nerves and other times it doesn't fully restore power to all of its parts.

Luckily, Quantum Neurology® has scientific ways to test the strength and weakness of different nerves. Once we know what is or is not working we can treat the individual nerve so that it can pass its messages along its wires properly. We'll get more into the details about how we do this in the next chapter.

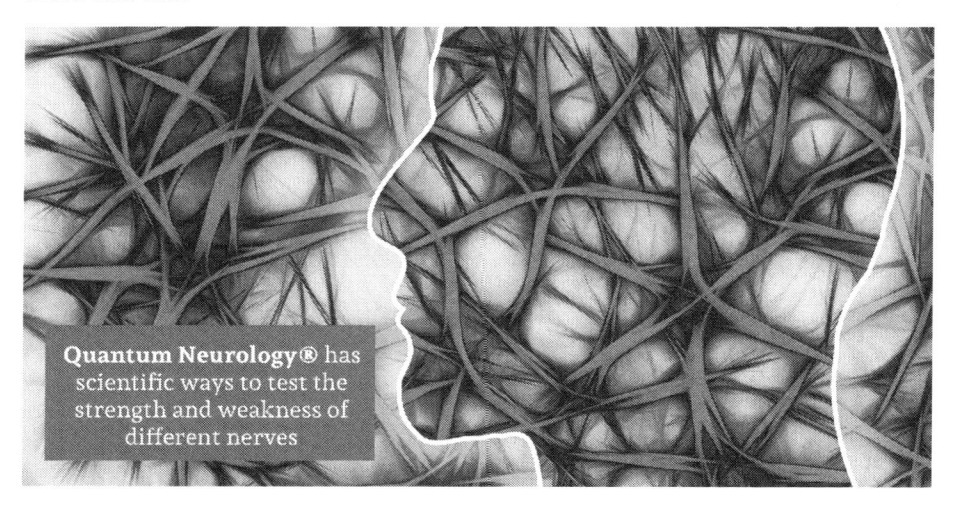

> **Quantum Neurology®** has scientific ways to test the strength and weakness of different nerves

Genetic components of wiring comes from Mom and Dad

Initially, everything about your body comes from your biological parents and ancestors. Whether you are tall or short, whether your eyes are blue or brown, and whether you are prone to certain diseases—all come from the genes that are passed to you by your mother and father.

We were all taught in basic biology class that you receive half of your genes from your mother via the egg and the other half from your father via the sperm. Your nervous system is the first thing that develops. It starts forming as soon as the sperm meets the egg. Nothing in your body can exist or function without a working nervous system.

Just like you may have inherited your father's nearsightedness or your mother's tendency toward arthritis, you may have inherited weak nerves from one or both of your parents. There isn't a whole lot you can do about genetics. What you've inherited from your parents is what you've inherited—you can't change that any more than you can change your height or the texture of your hair.

What you can do, however, is to check and maintain your body's top 3 ingredients with the OWL Method™. This gives your body the best chance to stay healthy and age more slowly. It also gives your body the ability to overcome bad genetics.

I'm a great example of this. My dad had his first back surgery when he was 19 years old. He had another back surgery in his thirties. The nerves in the lower back provide power to the muscles in the legs in addition to organs like the kidneys and pancreas. Over time, these nerves lost function and he developed diabetes. Proper care wasn't given to his nerves and he ended up having a pancreas and kidney transplant at 59 years old. Once you have any transplant, you are given heavy doses of immunosuppressants and can be more vulnerable to infections or sicknesses. Unfortunately, he died when he was just 67.

My back started out having problems at a very young age. I remember being in college and my back "going out" entirely, hardly being able to walk for days or weeks. This has happened dozens of times in my life, but fortunately I've been able to avoid surgeries or injections. Through proper nerve rehabilitation and the OWL Method™, my back is better now than it was in my twenties! It is possible to overcome bad genetics. My goal has always been to give the best genes possible to my current and future family.

HELPING OTHERS

The people I know who have a calling to help others (especially with zero expectation) tend to experience higher levels of fulfillment and live longer.

I asked myself if I could create that same opportunity to deliver this same value to you while you're reading this book.

So to do that, I have a question for you...

Would you help someone out that you've never met? Even if it didn't cost you a dime and you didn't get credit for it?

If that is the type of person you are, I have a huge ask from a man who grew up on a farm, and just wants to make the world healthier one person at a time.

There are people out there like you, who want to live healthier lives but are unsure to look... and this is where you come in.

The only way the Nerve Health Institute can achieve our vision of helping solve health's most difficult problems, is by first, reaching the right people.

With that being said, most people do in fact judge a book by its cover (and reviews)

So...

If you feel you have received any value from this book so far, would you do me a huge favor and leave an honest review of the book and even something you might have learned from it?

It will cost you a grand total of $0 and maybe about a minute of your time.

The impact of your review will impact...

...one more person dealing with difficult health challenges

...one more mother or father wanting to be alive and healthy enough to enjoy their future grandchildren.

...one more patient saved from the trappings and constraints of traditional medicine.

...one more life given years, maybe even decades of health back

...one more life changed for the better.

To have that level of impact and make that a reality, all you have to do is... leave a review.

PS – If you feel awesome about helping a person you may never meet, you are my kind of people.

PPS – Cool life hack: Introducing something valuable to someone, associates you with being someone of value. If you'd like to help others directly – send this book to them.

Thank you, from me to you, from the bottom of my heart.

Let's dive back in.

Your buddy, Dr. Chris.

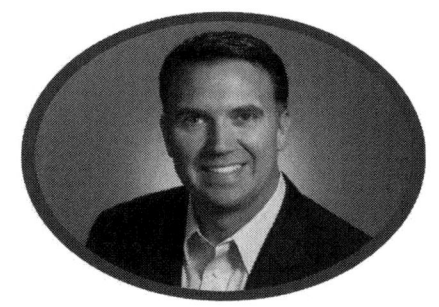

Chapter 3

The Nerve Breaker Box

Just like the electrical system in your house is regulated by the breaker box, there is a similar system in your body—the nerve breaker box. In the electrical system in your house, the breakers are tripped by a surge in electricity, which is a protective mechanism. When there is too much electricity surging through that particular set of wires, the breaker shuts off so that the amount of electricity doesn't overwhelm the system. When the breaker is tripped, you have to go and manually turn it back on, letting the system know it is okay to operate again.

Your body works in much the same way, only instead of a surge of electricity it would be a surge of light. Imagine that the power company in your body is your brain and spinal cord, which connects through nerves to every millimeter in your body. There aren't any human beings who have all millimeters of their bodies connected fully through light to the brain and spinal cord—everyone has power outages. The more power outages or breakers shut off, the more symptoms, illness, and disease you develop.

Power outages in the human body happen all the time depending on what you are doing, thinking about, breathing, eating, drinking, etc. Those days or times you feel not fully up to par are times when you have more power outages than is normal for you.

Because your body is a self-healing machine, sometimes it will reboot these power outages or turn back on these breakers, but sometimes it does not. This is the primary reason that some people age faster, get injured more easily, get more symptoms or get more illnesses or sicknesses than others.

Different stressors turn on and off nerves

Stress comes at different times and in many different forms throughout our entire lives:

1. Physical stress: this is posture, injuries (mild, moderate or severe), sports, activities, activities of daily living, etc.

2. Emotional stress: this is all the happenings in our lives causing conscious and subconscious thoughts to occur.

3. Biochemical stress: this is everything we eat, drink, breathe, and absorb.

These stressors can have temporary and sometimes lifelong consequences. To fully understand this, it's important to understand how your nervous system reacts to stress. You have two different nervous systems that operate automatically and involuntarily.

First, the sympathetic nervous system is your fight or flight reflex. It kicks in when something stressful happens. When it is in control, you feel anxious, or worried, or you might be on high alert. Your hands might be cold or you might be sweating. You might shake or your muscles might tense up. Many people's hearts beat more rapidly. This side of the nervous system needs a significant amount of light power.

Secondly, the parasympathetic nervous system helps you go to sleep. When it is in charge of your body, you can heal and rest. This is also when your body does its digesting and repairing. This side of the nervous system needs less light power.

When your body is reacting in a fight or flight manner, all of these parasympathetic activities get put on hold. Your body uses all its energies to stay focused on keeping you safe from whatever danger it perceives is threatening you. You don't want to stay too long in either state. You don't want to be in a place of high stress or complete rest at all times. It's best to be somewhere in the middle.

If you don't stay in the middle, stress hormones will trip those breakers we talked about a few pages ago. This causes your body to use up its light power. Lower light power means weaker nerves. The more stressors you have, the more those breakers are going back and forth in unnatural ways that prevent the ideal functioning of your body.

It's impossible to just prevent stress from happening. Life can and will be stressful at times. We worry about our jobs and our families and our health. If everyone knew about the OWL Method™, we would handle stress so much better.

Checking and maintaining the body's top 3 ingredients enables the body to stay healthier and more resilient to stress, injuries, illnesses or sicknesses.

By using the OWL Method™ and Quantum Neurology® we can get into the nervous system and assess weakness. We can go into your brain and spinal cord and every millimeter of your body and see where the weaknesses are happening. Everything is hardwired together. Nerves are fiber optic, so they use light. You don't want nerves to stay disconnected and have light power outages.

Likewise, we can make sure that you are properly hydrated. It might be as simple as drinking more water! We can give you concentrated oxygen with our hyperbaric oxygen chambers as well as exercise with oxygen therapy.

The goal is to stay closer to the middle between parasympathetic and sympathetic. We want to get your heart beating at a normal speed more consistently. We want you to use your fight or flight reflex and then go back to the middle. Too much fight or flight reflex causes our muscles to tense up and pull your bones, tendons, and ligaments out of alignment.

How we check the nerves

Because we have now been able to map the nervous system and all 88 nerves, we know where they go and what parts of the body they control. When you come into my office, I can test the strength or weakness of all the nerves in the body. When we are doing this testing, our patients can instantaneously feel these weaknesses as we are testing for them. Each time a nerve weakness is found, the brain begins trying to restore light power to the weakened part. If your brain doesn't know where light power outages are, it oftentimes won't ever restore these weaknesses.

Once we know which nerve isn't working properly, it's simply a matter of adding light power to that nerve to enable your body to heal itself better. Your body is made to heal itself. It is truly miraculous! All it needs is the space and materials to do it, and the lack of interference. This is where Quantum Neurology® comes in.

Quantum Neurology®

Quantum Neurology® was discovered by Dr. George Gonzalez. It's a method of making sure the nerves are working correctly, which allows us to operate as pain free and as healthy as possible. There aren't very many Advanced Quantum Neurologists in the world. I'm so proud to be one of the pioneers of this revolutionary rehabilitation technique.

This specialized and naturalized way of rehabilitating the body by focusing on the nervous system is both self-healing and preventative for literally everyone. In today's world, it is impossible to avoid neurological weaknesses. The brain has to have connections to all the parts in the human body. Sometimes we don't detect the problem before it causes a problem.

Quantum Neurology® is about keeping your nervous system as strong as possible at all times. When your nervous system is strong, there's very little that can overcome the power of the human body. Whenever your nervous system is functioning at less than 100 percent of its capability, you're setting yourself up for an injury or sickness.

In other words, the probability of injury is directly related to how strong your nervous system is. By resetting the "breaker box" for the body, you can greatly accelerate the body's ability to self-heal.

Certain postures that we put our bodies in might be tripping these breakers. It might be certain foods that we are eating, and genetics make us prone to have the breaker trip. We might have inherited a "faulty" breaker from one of our parents. All of these factors, plus so many more, might play into what is "on" and what is "off" in our breaker box.

There are a lot of factors involved in keeping your breakers on. The only way to know which breakers are on and which are off is to see someone like me who can test your nerves and see which ones are working. I can go into your breaker box and see where the wires are not signaling.

For example, if I take your hand and grip it, the muscles in your hand cause it to grip mine. We want the wiring signal or light power that is going from your brain to your hand to be firing very well. If that light-powered signal is slow, the grip is weaker than it should be, and you most likely have no idea (see *Hidden*

Diagnosis). There is a small group of us that have a much better understanding of this, who can find this hidden diagnosis and actually repair it. We're capable of going into the breaker box and repairing the individual breakers/nerves on a quantum level to make sure that you are working at your optimum to prevent and repair injuries.

Chapter 4

The *Hidden Diagnosis* in Elite Athletes

Elite athletes have a *hidden diagnosis* that is preventing them from taking their "game" to the next level. It lies within their nervous system and they don't even know it. Their doctors and trainers are missing it.

Did you know that your most prized asset as an elite athlete is your body's nervous system? The nervous system is the brain and everything that it connects to in the body: muscles, tendons, ligaments, organs, bones, etc. It's *not* muscles that move the feet, arms, legs or hands. It is the brain.

Without a wiring connection from your brain, a muscle will not work. If a signal from your brain to one or more of your muscles is not firing at 100 percent (the *hidden diagnosis*), the risk of injury drastically increases and the potential to maintain elite status drastically decreases. This is the deep-rooted reason why so many injuries are occurring even without any contact, e.g. tearing the anterior cruciate ligament (ACL).

I've treated many elite athletes who come to me saying, "I don't need help. My nervous system is strong because I can bench press 300+ pounds and squat 500+ pounds. My 40-yard dash time is 4.7 and my vertical jump is 36 inches." These athletes are completely dumbfounded when I show them hidden weaknesses within their nervous system. They are even more surprised after they see and feel those weaknesses get immediately corrected.

Fixing the *hidden diagnosis* is the "edge" that all elite athletes are looking for.

The biggest *hidden diagnosis* in elite athletes is weak brain connectivity to very important muscles in the knees, arms, shoulders, neck and back. Playing with these hidden weaknesses makes it very probable that you will be injured, stay injured or you will never reach your full potential as an elite athlete.

Let's look at some possible scenarios—ones in which weak nerves can result in very tangible losses:

- If one finger on a quarterback's hand isn't 100 percent connected to the brain, that finger is weaker than it should be, causing the quarterback's throws to be less accurate than they could be. Maybe he misses the game-winning touchdown throw by a foot because this finger has a *hidden diagnosis*. We can easily find and fix that.

- Here's another cool example. Planet Earth is filled with colors that we have to see, wear, eat, and breathe. Think about a team who gets intimidated and loses badly to another team year after year. Many times this is compounded by the players' *hidden diagnoses* (neurological weaknesses) to the color of the opposing team's jerseys and/or helmets. So when they prepare for the game and step onto the field, they see the color of the other team's jerseys and they start getting weak, without knowing or feeling it. So, as soon as they see the actual color of the opponent's uniform, breakers begin to trip in their breaker boxes. This is just like breakers tripping in your house. In this case, I find and strengthen the players' hidden weak nerves to the opposing team's jersey and/or helmet color. The results are amazing!

- Maybe you are trying to get your vertical jump higher or your 40-yard dash time faster—what if you have a *hidden diagnosis* in your starting position? We can find and fix that, which will improve your speed and jumping capabilities.

- Emotions and thoughts can also trigger nerve weaknesses. Take the quarterback who throws an interception and loses the game. Thereafter, every time he thinks about that interception, breakers start tripping in his brain and body. In the office, we would take actual footage from that interception and strengthen his nervous system while he's watching the video, so that if he's ever in that scenario again, about to throw the last pass of the game, the likelihood of him throwing an interception because of tripped breakers is much lower.

- As an elite athlete, you need to make sure that your brain is properly connected to the muscles in your eye so that you can move your eyes in all directions needed. Let's look at an elite baseball player, a great hitter can experience a six- month hitting slump. If he has a neurological weakness related to cranial nerve 6, which moves the eyes from side to side, every time he's setting up to bat and looking at a pitch, he's in a weakened neurological state. This is a major reason big-time hitters repeatedly fall into "slumps" whereby they go from hitting the ball every game to repeatedly striking out. A baseball player needs the connection from his brain—through the cranial nerves—into his eye to be strengthened before he can make the necessary corrections to his hitting.

I feel confident that the teams that win Superbowls, the World Series, and championships, as well as the individuals who win the Masters and other major sporting events, are all more neurologically sound, as a whole, than losing teams and individuals.

Another consideration is with the current alarming increase of football players' size and speed. It is becoming harder and harder for athletes to take repeated blows and get back up the next day, week or season. Twenty years ago, it seemed impossible that a 6'5" football player weighing 250 pounds would ever break 4.8 in the 40-yard dash, but in 2022, players of this size can run a 4.5! However, faster and bigger players are part of the reason why careers are ending and unforeseen injuries are oftentimes coupled with serious neurological injuries.

Getting hit by a 250-pound linebacker, who runs a 4.5 40-yard dash, is the equivalent of getting hit by an all-terrain vehicle traveling at 18 mph. As a football player, you will have to encounter hundreds of hits from players like this coming at all different angles to your body. Given these circumstances, how is it possible to have career longevity and at the peak of health? The answer is to protect the body's most valuable asset—the nervous system!

I recently treated an elite college football player who had torn his ACL the previous season and was gearing up to get back on the field. After reconstructive ACL surgery, he had gone through months of serious physical therapy to rehabilitate his knee. Upon my initial examination, all of the brain connections to his legs were rock solid, with the exception of one major muscle in his left leg. His left sartorius muscle, which is the muscle that pulls the foot across the body and simultaneously flexes the hip, was connected at less than 30 percent to his brain, and he had no idea. He barely had any strength when this muscle was resisted in his left leg, and this elite athlete had been cleared to play at 100 percent by all the other medical professionals and trainers assigned to his case. If he had started playing football again in that condition, he would have survived without further injury only out of sheer luck.

By using the new science of Quantum Neurology®, this athlete's brain's connection to his left leg was restored from 30 to 100 percent. He went from not being able to pull his foot across his body while flexing his knee to being rock-solid strong in seconds. This was taken a step further by figuring out and correcting why his brain had lost the signal into his left sartorius muscle in the first place. In other words, why had this signal turned off? In his case, every time he fully extended his neck (e.g. a routine tackle for a linebacker), the signal was turning off in his left leg. Subsequently, his leg was further strengthened with simultaneous resisted neck extension. These major corrections to his nervous system took place within a few visits, and when he returned to the football field for his senior college season, he was strong enough to avoid tearing his ACL again, in addition to having a much stronger neck.

Furthermore, I contend that this 6'3", 240-pound athlete had a *hidden diagnosis* prior to tearing his ACL. How else is it possible that a ligament the size of a dime in diameter could fully tear? Was it simply because this athlete was exerting too much force? No, it was because this athlete already had a *hidden diagnosis* in his leg before his injury. This is precisely why some people tear their ACLs and others don't.

Finding these hidden nerve weaknesses and strengthening them is the heart of Quantum Neurology®. I am so proud to be one of the pioneering, advanced quantum neurologists in the development of the most revolutionary nerve rehabilitation technique ever created.

Keeping your body in tip-top shape is incredibly hard while you maintain a grueling schedule of helmet thrashing. Undoubtedly, at some point in your career, you will suffer with some type of injury. If you have the same luck as a winner of the Powerball Lottery, then you will finish a very long career without any injuries at all. As an elite football player, experiencing injuries, from mild

to severe, has become as common as eating a hamburger. Keeping your nervous system as strong as possible at all times through nerve rehabilitation is essential. When your nervous system is strong, there is very little that can overcome the power of your amazing human body.

Training, practicing and playing with a nervous system that is functioning at 100 percent means it is almost impossible to get injured on the football field. Conversely, whenever your nervous system is functioning at less than 100 percent of its capability, it is the perfect set-up for a serious and even career-ending injury. The probability of injury is directly related to how strong your nervous system is.

The statistics on players ending their careers much earlier than anticipated because of injury are increasing. There is no need for that to happen—Quantum Neurology® can help. GET CONNECTED! Stay ahead of the game and competitors. Lower the probability of injury and, in the case of injury, choose the fastest route to recovery. Jump higher, run faster, and strengthen your nerves. Diagnosing and strengthening hidden weak brain-to-body connections is the future for creating elite athletes.

Finally, it is also imperative for elite athletes to maintain cellular Oxygen, our number one ingredient. All elite athletes should be routinely doing Hyperbaric Oxygen Therapy and Exercise With Oxygen Therapy. Keeping adequate Oxygen allows them to heal faster and stay stronger and healthier to maximize their potential.

In the big picture, if elite athletes do the OWL Method™, they will stay on the field longer and healthier which makes them more money! Athletes not doing these things oftentimes lose millions of dollars throughout their careers.

Chapter 5

Why are we OWL Deficient?

One of the main reasons why these breakers trip in our breaker box is because we are deficient with some of our oxygen, water, and light.

Why are we OWL deficient? It seems odd, when you consider that these resources are abundant and largely free. All we need to do to get oxygen is to breathe. Water flows freely out of taps in every building we enter. Light exists at the flick of a switch and is free outdoors all day every day. So how come we just can't get enough?

Food Supply

Much of our deficiency has to do with our food supply. Our food supply is no longer natural. For thousands of years, the concept of "farm-to-table" was the norm. Most people grew their own vegetables in their own backyards. Meat came from their own farm animals or from those of the neighborhood butcher. The thought of an out-of-season strawberry was inconceivable.

It's only recently that we've had the technology to import fruits and vegetables and other foods from long distances. Factory farming is a concept that is only about a hundred years old—just a blip in human history. But wait, there's more. Now we have genetic modifying or engineering (GMO) of crops, poisonous fertilizers, and the antibiotics and steroids that we feed farm animals.

All you have to do is grow a tomato in your backyard to know the difference. Take a bite out of a grocery store tomato and one that you've grown yourself, and you won't be able to believe they come from the same plant. They taste so incredibly different. In order to make tomatoes commercially viable, they are poisoned, picked before ripeness, and have the nutrients all but stripped from them.

Our bodies need a whole host of nutrients in order to work properly. We need vitamins and essential minerals in order to process fuel and run our complicated chemistry in the right way. We are told that we can make up for this by taking vitamin supplements (which can also be genetically modified), but then we take them in pill forms which don't involve the natural digestive process.

God made us to take in nutrients primarily through the food and drinks we consume—not through artificial chemicals or things packed into little pills. The mechanical and artificial manipulation of vitamins changes them so much that our bodies can't absorb them like we can if we get them through eating and drinking real God-made foods. Liquefied God-made foods, rather than lab-made pills, are far superior for your body. This is one of the reasons why I've developed supplements using natural food sources. See the resources section at the end for information on how to find them.

Environment

Our environment has become increasingly artificial. In the past hundred years, we've gone from being a largely agrarian society to one that works in hermetically sealed office buildings with recycled air and fluorescent lighting. We go from our air-conditioned offices to our air-conditioned cars to our air-conditioned houses.

All of this has consequences. We are rarely exposed to sunlight and all the benefits it has. We don't get the vitamin D we need from sunshine; instead we have to get it from infused milk and dairy products, which are also infused with antibiotics and hormones. We no longer walk any further than from the door to our car, and even that is inside a parking garage most of the time.

Because we don't walk (or ride horses) for transportation anymore, we drive cars, which belch carbon monoxide and smog into the air. So in addition to the oxygen and carbon dioxide and helium and all the natural clean elements that we breathe in, we are also breathing in pollutants which interfere with our body's ability to make use of the oxygen we need to live.

We're busy people. We don't have time or energy to tend our gardens, if we have them, and agriculture is a largely automated big business. Farmers don't go out every day to weed their crops and pull harmful insects off the leaves by hand. Instead, it's easier to grow genetically modified crops that are resistant to certain pests, or to spray weed killers that are designed to kill the weeds but not the genetically modified plants the farmers want. Machines that use fossil fuels pick the crops, and then spray them with more poison to preserve them, then wrap them in plastic.

There are so many chemicals involved, and good, clean dirt is virtually nonexistent. The plants that compost are not exactly organic material. The chemicals that have been sprayed on them contaminate the soil and the groundwater. All of this gets picked up by the plants that grow through their roots, and the livestock when they eat the plants and drink the water. Finally, we consume all these toxins when we eat meat, fruits, and vegetables.

This interferes with our body's ability to function properly. It's hard to get the right balance of vitamins and minerals when you are ingesting things you were never meant to ingest. Your body isn't sure what to do with these toxins or genetically modified things. They are one of many stressors on your nervous system, and as a result, some of the breakers in your breaker box turn off.

It's almost impossible in modern times to remove toxins completely from your diet and your environment, but you can do your best by avoiding genetically modified foods, eating organically grown fruits and vegetables when possible, drinking purified water, getting as much sunshine and light as you can, eating farm-to-table or locally grown foods, and supplementing your diet with natural, non-lab-processed supplements like the ones I've recommended in the resources section at the end of this book.

You can also make sure that your indoor air is healthier. About 85 percent of American adults spend their time indoors, breathing in polluted air. Oxygen is our #1 nutrient but what else are we breathing? Carbon monoxide? Pesticides? Molds? Bacteria? Viruses? Parasites? Many cleaning sprays and solutions are also very toxic. Indoor air can undermine our health.

I often invent things for my own family's health that end up having value for my patients. More than 8 years ago I started realizing I had a lot of sick people coming into my office and I decided I needed to change the quality of indoor air. I realized that plants have essential oils that they emit as a protective layer, and which have antimicrobial properties—it's what the plant uses to prevent predators from hurting them. I made a formula based on 4 ingredients that have different properties and benefits—lemongrass, clove, cinnamon bark, and peppermint oil. That oil, which we had tested at the University of Louisiana at Lafayette, killed all kinds of microbes. I call it Oil2Air®.

Unfortunately, and despite having official documents from the university proving what it kills, the FDA has a clause with policies not allowing any essential oils to be classified as drugs. It is for this reason that we can't make claims, even though we have the real proof from the chief microbiologist.

Furthermore, I invented an Oil2Air® diffuser that hooks onto the return air vent where your air filter is. The air, as it circulates, continually distributes the oil throughout all the vents in your house. So every day, as your HVAC is working, the antimicrobial properties of the essential oils are working. It also smells great! To find out where you can get Oil2Air®, see the resources section at the end.

Chapter 6

Healing Without DIS (Drugs, Injections, and Surgery)

There's an old saying that goes, "When you're a hammer, everything looks like a nail." So when you go to a surgeon, everything looks like it needs surgery. When you go to a medical doctor, every problem looks like it needs to be solved with drugs or injections.

I'm not saying that drugs, injections, and surgery don't have their place. Sometimes they are necessary, but not all the time—not even most of the time they are recommended. Before you take these drastic actions, you have to give the body a chance to heal itself.

Teaching the body to heal itself

The body is remarkably good at healing itself. In fact, if we do too much to artificially heal it using outside means, we can do more harm than good. Ear infections, for example, are most likely to go away on their own. Antibiotics don't do much to help them, even though many doctors are so quick to prescribe them. This can do more harm than good, since prescribing antibiotics too much often creates "superbugs" that are antibiotic resistant, and then the antibiotics don't work when you do need them. That's just one example of how it can be a bad thing to refuse to let the body heal itself when it is perfectly capable of doing so.

Before you resort to drugs, injections, or surgery, do what you can to heal naturally. Give your body the tools it needs to heal on its own. Make sure you are not oxygen, water or light deficient. See a professional like me who can help you and who can teach you at-home exercises that will help your body heal.

At-home exercises

When people come to see me, I can give them a lot of relief. That makes me happy, and it's why I love my job. But I know there's only so much relief I can give them in my office. They can only come in so often, and what happens between sessions matters. It's important that my patients and everyone following me learns how to do some things at home so that they can keep up the nerve strength we've achieved. It's all part of teaching the body how to heal itself.

I'm not a big fan of rest. When it comes to things in your body with pain, it starts with neurological weakness. Rest further atrophies your muscles and nerves. You have to make the brain fire those parts that aren't working to get them sparked back up. This is the only way to get your power back and start to do the things you want to do.

Below, I'll describe a couple of my more popular recommendations for people to attain and maintain strength to help with some common complaints.

Examples

Back Pain

Many people come to me complaining of pain in their back and in their legs. This simple exercise will help if you feel any pressure

Healing Without DIS (Drugs, Injections, and Surgery)

or pain in your back. It's a way to preemptively strike back and prevent future flare-ups.

For this exercise, take a flat pillow of any kind—a couch pillow will do.

While standing, place the pillow between your knees and do a little squat. Make sure all your weight is on your heels. All you are doing is squatting backward. The easiest way to think of this position is if you are camping and you have to go to the bathroom in the woods. You want to get your butt as far away from your feet as you can without falling down. If you want to do it in front of a wall, but without touching the wall with your butt, so you have that safety net, that's fine. Keep squeezing the pillow between your legs, and shift your weight from left to right, back and forth, back and forth. Your weight should be in your heels the whole time.

Do that for about 30 seconds, and then come back up and see how it feels. If it makes you feel a little better, then do it again. Discontinue if for any reason it worsens your pain.

While you are doing this exercise, the muscles at the top of your butt should feel like they are getting their power back. The muscles on the top of your thighs are also engaging and getting their power back. This is a wonderful exercise for people who have weak backs. So many people have recurrent episodes and a family history of their backs "giving out". Maybe you have a history where your relatives have had back surgery and a weak back has passed from generation to generation. Even with this family history, you can help strengthen these nerves and muscles and help avoid the family curse. Practice this to save yourself from history.

Sleep

You can sleep in a way that helps your nerves operate better.

You want all of your 88 nerves to stay powered on as well as possible, especially when you sleep. Your body should rest and heal while you are sleeping and you should wake up refreshed. It's important to sleep in a way that keeps your body well aligned.

Sleep positions are critical. So many of my patients ask what the best position is to sleep in that will maintain their nerve health. Remember, your brain and spinal cord are at the top, and all 88 nerves branching off from them power up everything else in your body. When you sleep you should be relaxed and wake up feeling great. So many people wake up feeling stiff and sore. This means they are doing things in their sleep that are not right.

In a perfect world, people would have a bed with a hole for their faces so they could lie face down in a nice, comfortable, relaxed position. Unfortunately, no one has a bed like that. So many people try to sleep on their bellies, and that isn't good. They turn their heads, kink up their arms and shoulders, and bend up a knee. All the vertebrae have to be turned and the spinal cord has to be turned and twisted. The shoulders are rotated upward and outward. The vertebrae by the ribs are twisted, which can affect your lungs and breathing.

People will also sleep with one leg propped up to one side. That will twist the lower back, called the lumbar or sacrum. It can diminish blood flow down to one leg versus the other. Of all the positions you can sleep in, this is the worst, yet there are so many people doing it—laying on the belly, neck twisted, hips askew.

The pillow makes it worse. The pillow is too high, so you are bent back, which jams things even more. You are going to have problems if you sleep on your belly over time.

So here are some other positions which are much better for you. Sleeping on your back is a good position. But if you do, make sure your pillow is very narrow. You want the neck to be curved backward a little bit. You don't want your neck bent forward, otherwise you might wake up with numbness in the arms and a

stiff neck. If your arms are above your head, you might wake up with numbness or tingling in your hands because of decreased blood flow to your hands or nerve problems. Your arms and hands should be by your sides.

The idea is that you want to keep your nerve health good at night so that your body can heal. You don't need to be military and stiff, but you want to keep your body relatively straight. You could be on your side with your knees bent. For this position, you want to make sure your pillow is not too low so that your neck doesn't bend down. The pillow has to accommodate the width from your mattress to your ear. Some people prefer to put something between their knees. You don't want to rotate your pelvis.

In a nutshell, you want to be on your side or on your back. Maintain some symmetry in your body. If you wake up every morning hurting, stiff, or numb, you're doing something wrong. You should wake up feeling rested and relaxed, ready to tackle what you need to do during the day.

Headache or Eye Strain

We've all felt eye strain, where you feel pressure or strain behind your eyes or around your eyebrows. This is a simple exercise you can do to help alleviate that discomfort. Put a little bit of counter pressure on your eyeball. Start on one side—don't do both eyes at once to start. Make sure not to use too much pressure. Please don't hurt yourself or force anything. Use just a little pressure on your eyeball. While you do that, look up and look down, then look left and right. You might find a certain spot that relieves some of the pain that you have in this area.

Of course, make sure your hands are clean. You carry a lot of dirt and germs on your hands, and your eyes can easily transfer that dirt and germs into your system. So wash your hands before you start.

When you're done, do the other eyeball. Obviously, if it makes anything hurt more, stop what you're doing. But you'll likely be surprised how much relief you get. It helps to restore the sense of pressure to the cranial nerves providing power to your eyes. When these nerves get weak to pressure, it can make the eye get this headache-type feeling.

This is a simple little exercise you can do anywhere and anytime. Practice it when you get headaches or eyestrain and you may find a great deal of relief.

Vertigo

Balance is a great thing, but it can be dangerous if you lose the ability to control it.

We live on a planet that has a force that is pulling us downward. When you can no longer balance, that force—gravity—is going to cause you to potentially fall.

You are wired in a way that means you have different nerves powering up different muscles to enable you to balance—if you can't raise a foot up and balance on one leg, that's not good. You also have a pair of nerves inside your skull called cranial nerve 8, or the vestibular cochlear nerve. Vestibular means "balance" and cochlear means "hearing", and this same nerve enables you to both balance and hear.

Balance is also helped by seeing your surroundings through your ocular nerves. Making sure these balancing and seeing nerves are working together greatly helps our patients with vertigo or balance problems.

Practicing the following exercise helps with something called your vestibulo-ocular reflex whereby you mesh your ocular nerve with your vestibular nerve. Put your finger about a foot in front of you, directly in front of your nose. Focus on your fingertip. Bend your head forward and backward while keeping your focus on your fingertip. Then turn your head to the left and right, all the while keeping your focus on your fingertip. Now, tilt your head to the left and right, maintaining focus on your fingertip. What we see a lot of times is that people move their eyes. This won't work if you don't keep your focus. This exercise will help tremendously with your balance and your focus.

Doing this simple exercise can help to keep you on your feet and prevent falls. For more tips and home exercises to help with various conditions, please see the resources page at the end of this book where you can get access 24 hours per day to our Membership page with all of our proprietary exercises and methods to help various conditions at home.

Chapter 7

What can we do at Home?

In addition to the exercises I described in Chapter 5, there are so many other things you can do at home. You can make sure that the foods you eat are conducive to your health, and you can make sure that you are connected to the Earth.

Purity of foods

We've talked a little bit in Chapter 4 about the lack of purity in our food supply. The old saying is true, "You are what you eat." Your food is not just fuel for your body, but it is the raw material that your body uses to create new cells. If you are giving your body inferior or toxic building materials, then the cells your body creates with those building materials are themselves going to be inferior or toxic.

Furthermore, don't discount the value of putting quality fuel into the miraculous machine that is your body. Your body consists of several trillion cells, all of which have to function together smoothly in order for things to work properly. If they don't have good fuel, it isn't going to work. If even one cell doesn't have the right fuel, it will break the communication chain and the message isn't going to be passed on in the right way.

That's why it's important to ensure that we eat foods that are as pure as possible. Avoid processed foods. If you can't pronounce the ingredients on the label of what you're eating, you shouldn't be eating it.

What you want are organic, *whole* foods. You don't want foods where part of the nutrients has been stripped away. Whole foods are natural foods, meaning they exist exactly as God made them, from the earth and taken directly from nature. They have amino acids, vitamins, minerals, enzymes, and all kinds of other nutrients in perfect ratios that your body needs in order to function in the right way.

Most Americans have a poor diet. They don't eat enough fruits and vegetables, and the ones they do eat have been denaturalized. They're soaked in pesticides and preservatives; they've been canned, frozen, packaged, and processed. It is a rare American who regularly eats a simple, organically grown fruit or vegetable every day.

Take aloe vera—it is something that is easy to grow and easy to find. It has a myriad of health benefits. It works externally to help repair your skin, and it works internally to help a number of conditions like diabetes, asthma, epilepsy, and osteoarthritis. You don't need to do anything to aloe vera to make it work—just ingest the inner gel of the plant.

So many companies try to sell man-made versions of this wonderful plant. Aloe products should only be prepared by hand. Instead, you get machine-processed aloe, dehydrated, pasteurized, and otherwise processed aloe. Something so simple is made so complicated, and by over-complicating it, it is made less effective, with fewer nutrients in the proper ratios as God intended.

Synthetic supplements are not helpful

As a result, the vitamin supplement industry has become enormous. People are aware that they aren't getting the nutrients they need and so, typically lazy, they want a magic pill to fix everything. The supplement industry obliges.

Your body was not designed to digest pills, it was designed to digest food and liquids. Pure, natural food and drink in their simplest forms. Pills are probably the least natural forms of nutrients you can find. In 23 years of looking at X-rays of thousands of my patients, I often see undigested vitamin pill-shaped tablets in the lower digestive tracts. This means that the pills had done nothing but travel, mostly intact, through my patients' systems with virtually no absorption.

If you eat an apple, your body knows what to do with that apple. If you eat spinach, your body knows what to do. If you eat a man-made synthetic capsule, your body has no idea what to do with it, and it can reject it.

For some reason, we've got this idea that man-made things are better than God-made things. Somehow, we think the potassium we create in a lab and cram into a pill is better than the potassium we get from a banana, in perfect ratio with so many other nutrients. Despite all the sophistication in food science labs, scientists still haven't figured out the ingredients in a pear or an orange. We can't duplicate that magic formula in a lab. Why would we want to, when all that perfection grows on a tree?

There are a number of superfoods we can eat that provide a vast array of nutrients that give a supercharge to our bodies. These are all natural, grown-in-the-earth plants. They are foods like acai berries, goji berries, mangosteen, pomegranate, blueberries, peaches, pears, grapes, and green tea. I blend them together in a liquid formula called Superfruits GT for my patients to drink at

What can we do at Home?

home. Since it is a liquid formula, it's as close to the natural form of the fruits as you can find in a bottle.

There are also some wonderful superfoods like aloe vera, pau d'arco, cranberry, and white grape. The perfect whole food liquid blend of these is a supplement called SeaAloe. We have taken it for over 19 years now.

If you'd like some Superfruits GT or SeaAloe, or more recommendations and information, check out the resources section at the end of this book.

Connection to the Earth

We are so insulated from real life these days. We cover ourselves with clothing and chemicals that "protect" us from the Earth and from sunshine. True, those "protections" keep harmful insects and cancer-causing UV rays away from our skin, but they also keep all the benefits of the natural Earth away from us as well.

The Earth is naturally magnetically charged. The North Pole and the South Pole are not geographical markers, but magnetic ones. When you use a compass, the compass finds north based on a magnetic charge that is always present. That magnetic charge is natural and God-made and beneficial to your health overall and the health of your cells in particular.

The Superhuman Protocol

We're not far removed from our ancestors, running outside with hardly any clothes on and wearing no shoes. Since they were barefoot, they were touching the Earth when they walked outside.

Planet Earth also used to have a lot less pollutants and a lot more oxygen in the air. So, in essence, if you were outside, your bare feet would be touching the Earth, and the planet would be giving your body a magnetic charge. This would charge your cells giving slightly more alkalinity. You were also getting wonderful sunlight without light-blocking clothing. You weren't sitting in an office breathing indoor air, with your feet on concrete, and with your shoes blocking the magnetic charge.

Indoor air isn't full of clean oxygen. Often, there are harmful particles in indoor air. It isn't natural. Outside is generally healthier. There's more oxygen in the air.

Of course, it isn't reasonable to walk around naked, with your bare feet on the ground, breathing in good, clean oxygen for an hour or so a day. That's not something you can do in modern society. In the summer, you can walk barefoot with shorts and a T-shirt on, but you can't do that all the time. Even if this was possible, planet Earth has changed dramatically over the years. There is far less oxygen and more chemicals and pollutants in outdoor air. Planet Earth is less charged magnetically, and the sun has more harmful rays. It's hard to maintain these 3 basic ingredients of magnetism, oxygen and light.

This is why we have the Superhuman Protocol. Currently, there are a small number of clinics in the world that are certified to do the Superhuman Protocol, and I'm proud to be part of one of them. To find out how to locate the closest one to you, check out the resources section at the end.

With the Superhuman Protocol, you lie on a special mat that has the same magnetic charge as planet Earth. Instead of walking around barefoot, you can just lie on this mat. When you do that, your cells get charged. Your pH gets better, and your blood vessels open up. All of this happens in just 8 minutes.

Once you've done that, you do our Exercise with Oxygen Therapy—we call it EWOT. You have a mask that seals around your face with a giant tube that comes out of the middle. The tube is fed by a big bag that contains 94 percent oxygen. You are actually exercising with highly concentrated 94 percent oxygen, versus 21 percent oxygen in the air. You do that for up to 15 minutes.

After that, you lie unclothed in a private room on our TheraLight 360, so-called because it has 45,000 lights that reach every cell of your body. You do that for 10 minutes.

The whole Superhuman Protocol takes about 40 minutes. It's powerful—one of the most powerful things you can do to reset your oxygen and your light.

When we talk about oxygen, water, and light—the OWL Method™ of healthcare—it's about resetting your oxygen and light. It's really simple. Combine that with drinking enough clean water to hydrate your body, and your body will be able to heal itself, just as God intended.

Chapter 8

Success Stories with the OWL Method™

It's one thing for me to tell you how successful I've been with the OWL Method™ but it's another thing for my patients to give their own testimony. You can look at the Nerve Health Institute®'s channel on YouTube and find dozens and dozens of testimonials given by patients who have found near-instant relief from these methods. These simple things—oxygen, water, and light—have provided so much relief for so many suffering people.

In this book, I'd like to give you a few stories that will hopefully inspire you to seek out more. If you want to watch more of my videos, including testimonials, more exercises you can do at home, and informational videos, go to my YouTube channel here: https://www.youtube.com/channel/UC-XjChCw_Vx3Oa6s3TrEpYA

Story 1—Jennifer Cope

Jennifer Cope came into our office as a 32 year old woman in a wheel chair completely paralyzed from the waist down and unable to drive, walk, and take care of herself and her family. She had been in a wheelchair for over three months mainly due to a buildup of conditions caused by multiple sclerosis. Her dad begged her to come in and scheduled her an appointment after hearing about us from someone else at a gas station. Jennifer was very skeptical at first and thought that we were not going to be able to help her.

Her skepticism came to an end on just her second visit when after specific nerve health restoration, she got up out of the wheelchair and started walking! Upon driving back to her town, she became an immediate local celebrity and crowds of people were just absolutely amazed by what had happened. She has been walking fine now for almost 10 years!

The following quote is a direct quote from Mrs. Cope:

> "WOW... how you have changed my life and thanks to your amazing work I have been able to share my amazing testimony, about how you healed me and how you are continuously helping me and my family and friends, with so many people. You have no idea how many people just stop me in the grocery store or at the post office or gas station and just say "wow last time I saw you, you were in a wheelchair and that broke my heart. What new medication are you on?" I love getting to say that I was blessed to find this amazing Dr. in Lafayette who truly worked a miracle in my life! Of course, I give them your name and number because if they are not in need of your services they might know someone who is.
>
> Words cannot tell you how thankful I am for all that you do, not only am I thankful for how you have given me my life back but I am so thankful for how truly dedicated you are to your work and to your patients. I can see how honored you are to be able to help people and I can see that you don't look at this as a job, you enjoy every part of what you do!
>
> I truly consider you as my angel that God has put on this Earth and that God had truly led you to do what you are doing to help others live a healthier life and I am so grateful that we have crossed paths. I will continue to share my testimony about how my faithfulness in God kept me going and with answered prayers, along my journey, God led me to find you!

Thank you from the bottom of my heart for all that you do, please continue to strive to do more and I will continue to spread the word of your great works.
May God Bless You & Yours, Jennifer S. Cope"

Story 2—Tad Touchet

I got a text from Tad's dad saying that his son was in very bad health.

Tad was a very active young dad and husband in his twenties who was very involved in the family's car repair business and racehorse transportation business. A year before calling me, his lower back "gave out", and he experienced leg pain and sciatica with numbness and tingling. He saw a surgeon who recommended and performed surgery on his back. After a few months, there was no relief and symptoms were worsening. The same surgeon recommended another back surgery. A few months after performing this second surgery, Tad wasn't any better and his symptoms were worsening. The same surgeon recommended another back surgery. After performing the third back surgery in less than a year, his symptoms were worsening to the point where he was using a walker to walk. He couldn't sleep in his bed. He couldn't drive. He couldn't take care of himself, much less his wife or young daughter. He was very depressed. His life was spiraling downward at a fast pace.

After just a few months of seeing us for the OWL Method™, Tad has been fully back in the family business for almost 1 year now. He is walking, driving, traveling, sleeping and all the things a young man should be able to do. He is now driving massive trucks pulling racehorses all over the country. Most importantly, he is able to be the dad, husband and provider that he wants to be.

Story 3—Katrina McDaniels

Katrina was a 3-sport athlete in college. She got married and had a beautiful baby girl. Her life was that of many aspiring young families.

In October 2020, her life took a major turn. She was involved in an automobile crash that rendered her paralyzed from the chest down. After being hospitalized and going through many tests, doctors discovered she had suffered a life-spiraling-downward combination of a traumatic brain injury (TBI), a transient ischemic attack (TIA), and a spinal cord injury. Doctors gave her no hope and offered only a slew of medications with no likely possibility of walking again. She was just 25 years old and paralyzed with no feeling from her chest and core down into her legs. After many prayers, she was called to go to the Nerve Health Institute®.

In just 3 months of treatments with the OWL Method™ in our office, she was walking by herself—unassisted! She has been walking and functional for more than 1 year now. She is working her way up the ranks in her job and sometimes having to lift items over 70 lbs!

Katrina states, "Dr. Chris Cormier is the most compassionate, passionate and hardworking chiropractor I've ever known. He strives to fix—not to "cover up" (with meds, braces or surgeries) like my previous doctors."

Story 4—Griffin Hebert

During a football game, as a wide receiver, Griffin was running across the field and forcefully collided heads with a member of the opposing team. He instantly acquired a headache and had the "breath knocked out of him." He was brought immediately to the sidelines, showing both pupils dilated. He was benched from play for 2 weeks to follow the "concussion protocol".

Three weeks following the trauma, he was still experiencing concussion symptoms. He presented to the Nerve Health Institute® with headaches and extreme light sensitivity. It was determined that 5 of Griffin's 12 cranial nerves were dysfunctional. After a week of nerve rehabilitation, Griffin reached full resolution of his symptoms. He is back on the field and playing at 100 percent. He also finished his high school career and played an additional 5 years in college at Louisiana Tech Football.

Story 5—Gabe Lebeouf

Gabe was a great running back until he injured his shoulder in the beginning of his junior season in high school. He saw doctors who recommended that for the rest of his junior season, he wear a restrictive brace on his shoulder and only play linebacker (not running back). They recommended that after the football season they would do exploratory surgery on his shoulder to try to figure out the problem.

Thank goodness, Gabe and his family heard about us. He came to see us immediately following his junior season, and we found and repaired plenty of nerve weaknesses. He played his entire senior year as a starting running back and ended up winning the state championship. He never had surgery on his shoulder and is now in medical school.

Success Stories with the OWL Method™

Story 6—Will Tolson

At 10 years old, Will was a normal kid playing sports and having fun. Unfortunately, one day proved to be one of the worst for him. He was playing football for the Swampcats and during a game, took a small hit. Within minutes, he started to develop numbness and tingling throughout his body. They rushed him to the hospital (just 1/8 mile away) and by the time they arrived, he was paralyzed. The doctors ran scans and tests and really didn't give any explanation as to what was truly happening with him. They recommended that he see a neurosurgeon, who recommended mild physical therapy.

Luckily, they heard about us and decided to come in to see us. We were able to find and restore power to many nerve weaknesses in his body. He went from being paralyzed to running in just 2 visits! His mom, a neurosurgery nurse, was very skeptical, but was completely blown away at what we were able to do for her son in such a short period.

Story 7—Mason Patin

In the end of 2019, Mason got a virus and within a few days, he was paralyzed. He had severe pain in nearly every part of his body and couldn't tolerate even the slightest movement. His parents brought him to multiple doctors and clinics and hospitals and ultimately he was diagnosed with amplified musculoskeletal pain syndrome (AMPS).

Luckily, his parents heard about us and got him to see us. Since his second visit, he has been running! His life has dramatically changed for the better. He is now a fully functional young man.

Story 8—Rusty Noel

Football coach/founder of the Lafayette Swampcats.

While pulling on a large overhead pipe wrench, Rusty lost his grip, causing the pipe to strike him on the frontal portion of the skull, instantly dropping him to his knees.

He immediately experienced nausea, loss of balance, stiffened neck, arm tingling, buzzing/acute ringing in the ears, light sensitivity, and inability to drive.

He presented to the Nerve Health Institute® 2 days following the incident. First, we determined that he had a fractured skull. After a CT scan showed normal, without any brain bleed, we evaluated the functionality of the cranial nerves. It was determined that 6 of his 12 cranial nerves were dysfunctional. One of the alarming findings indicated he was unable to focus and was seeing 5 fingers when looking at just one finger.

After 9 treatments of nerve rehabilitation, Rusty reached full resolution of his symptoms. He never skipped a day of work throughout his nerve health restoration!

Story 9—Morgann Leleux Romero, Olympian Pole Vaulter

Morgann has been a patient for over 10 years. We have helped her overcome so many injuries and have watched her go from amateur to professional to Olympian! One of our proudest accomplishments with her has been keeping her in tip-top shape and preventing injuries and surgeries. Despite a torn labrum in her shoulder, we have helped her compete to her maximum capacity at the highest level.

Success Stories with the OWL Method™

This is a quote from Morgann about having me as her doctor after she became an Olympian: "Oh my goodness, oh my goodness, thank you so much for absolutely everything!!! You were such a gift from God!! And I could not have done this without you!!!!"

Throughout her athletic career, she has done all of our treatments and technologies... Nerve Health restoration and maintenance, Hyperbaric Oxygen Therapy, Superhuman Protocol, etc.

Story 10—Carmen Jefferson

I'm seeing a lot of patients now who have recovered—or, I should say partially recovered—from lung diseases. Carmen Jefferson is one of them. She was taking all kinds of vitamins as preventatives, but got sick anyway. She did okay for a few days, and then her oxygen levels dropped. She went to the Emergency Room, where she had a contrast CT scan and they found damaged lungs. She felt like she wasn't getting any care, so she left. She found an urgent care that treated her more naturally. She got inhalers and antibiotics and other drugs and oxygen. When she thought she was over it, her back was killing her and she couldn't breathe again. She came to see me this time. After I performed some tests on her, I realized the disease had weakened the nerves to her heart, lungs, kidneys, and pituitary glands. We restored fiberoptic light power from her brain to these organs and glands. I suggested the hyperbaric oxygen chamber, and she got instant relief. I suggested the Contour Light as well, and she got further relief from that too. She keeps repeating the hyperbaric chamber, and every time she gets more and more relief. She is so much better!

Story 11—Elaine

Elaine started the Superhuman Protocol to treat her COPD. She would get short of breath pretty easily. Since she began the protocol, she has a lot more stamina. She finds she has more energy and coughs a whole lot less. Before her treatment, she used to cough a lot in the morning to clear her lungs, and that has lessened, and during the day she coughs significantly less.

Story 12—Daniel

Daniel was skeptical of the Superhuman Protocol, but after only a week he noticed a difference. Daniel is a skater, and for 20 years, every time he wakes he's stiff and hurting. He drinks his coffee and tries to loosen up. Since he's been doing the Superhuman Protocol, he doesn't hurt at all. He especially thinks that EWOT helps him keep his energy and stamina.

Conclusion

Hopefully, you've learned that <u>our nervous system is basically a power station for our body. The nerves themselves are the breaker box for that power station. When one of the breakers gets shut off, everything that feeds from that nerve isn't going to get the messages it needs to do its job.</u>

Like all power stations, our nerves and the cells they are connected to in our bodies need light power to make them work properly. They also can't work properly if they don't have the right nutrients to feed them. They need the raw materials to build new cells and pass along all the messages through the nervous system. This comes from proper nutrition and the 3 most essential ingredients: oxygen, water, and light.

By using the OWL Method™ we can make sure that we have cured our bodies of their basic OWL deficiencies. We can fill our bodies with oxygen, pure water, and the right kind of light. We can reconnect with the Earth and its magnetic charge, eat natural foods, and keep ourselves hydrated and oxygenated.

Doing these simple things gives so many major benefits. Aside from simply feeling better, we can position our bodies to do what they were designed to do: heal themselves. Our bodies are miraculous machines. They have the ability to fix themselves when they are broken. But in order to do so, they have to have the right tools and raw materials.

<u>Only when our bodies have sufficient oxygen, water, and light will they have the ability to heal themselves to the highest potential.</u>

The result will be a lack of chronic aches and pains, general good health, and a shorter recovery time from injuries.

What are you waiting for? Get oxygen, water, and light today!

We now have a membership page for people who want to "Feel Better Fast At Home. On this membership page, you will have exclusive access to specific exercises that will help address specific conditions immediately. For example, if you have sinusitis, we will show you some exercises to turn nerves back on to your sinuses or enjoy some of our other natural protocols that you can do. It will be constantly updated. If you are interested in membership, please visit https://www.feelbetterfastathome.com

Resources

Full Spectrum Lights

Full spectrum lights are easy to find. You can get them at almost any big box store or online retailer. They are not all created equally, however. I recommend the Sauna Space light. Go to https://sauna.space/products

Hyberbaric Oxygen Treatment (HBOT)

As more people recognize the benefits of HBOT, it is becoming more widely available. You can find HBOT in your area by searching "HBOT" with your zip code or city. Please make sure you look for hard chambers (soft chambers only go up to 1.3 ATA which is considered "Mild HBOT").

Exercise with Oxygen Therapy (EWOT) *HOTB Burton*

You can find EWOT in your area by searching for Exercise with Oxygen Therapy with your zip code or city.

Salt Recommendations

Giants' flesh

~~Original Himalayan Salt is the best salt in the world~~, and can be bought exclusively through my own brand, Healthy Cajun™. Geaux2Salt and Geaux2Seasoning can both be bought at www.healthycajun.com/collections/all

Oil2Air®

To purchase any of our products like our essential oils, diffuser, or sprays, go here: https://oil2air.com

Quantum Neurologists

Quantum Neurology® is a relatively new field and, as of the writing of this book, there are only a few dozen quantum neurologists in the United States. You can find out if one is near you by visiting https://quantumneurology.com/find-a-quantum-neurology-doctor/

Be advised that quantum neurologists are trained in how to properly identify and fix neurological weaknesses and anyone not properly trained in Quantum Neurology® may not be giving you the treatment that will help you feel better fast.

SeaAloe/Superfruits GT

Superfruits GT is my formula and it is the most powerful SUPERFRUIT antioxidant combination in the world! It combines Resvератrol and Green Tea with 8 incredible superberries and fruits to create the ultimate antioxidant formula. It contains 11 of the world's best whole foods including Açai Berries, Mangosteen, Wolfberries, Pomegranate, Blueberries, Peaches, Pears, Luo Han Guo, White Grapes, Green Tea and Resveratrol.

SeaAloe is a powerful combination 13 of the world's best whole foods including 7 Sea Vegetables, Aloe Vera, Pau D'Arco, Cranberries, Black Cherries, White Grapes, and Concord Grapes. SeaAloe gives your body over 80 Vitamins, Minerals, Macro-Minerals, Trace Minerals, Phytonutrients, and all the Essential Amino Acids.

Resources

You can get SuperfruitsGT and SeaAloe here: https://naturesliquids.com

Superhuman Protocol

To find a clinic that is certified to use the Superhuman Protocol near you, check out https://appx.superhumanhp.com/locations

Water

To ensure that your water is pure, you can purchase a purification system for your entire home: https://www.davincimedicalusa.com/alkaviva-whole-home

You will need a certified plumber to install this technology.

About the Author

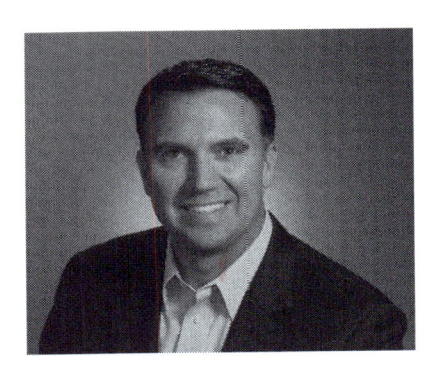

Dr. Chris Cormier graduated from Louisiana State University in 1994 with a Bachelor's Degree of Science in Kinesiology. He continued his education at Texas Chiropractic College in Houston, where he was a member of the Omega Psi Honors Fraternity and received his Doctorate of Chiropractic with Honors in 1998. Dr. Cormier is a licensed Chiropractic Physician in Louisiana and a member of the Chiropractic Association of Louisiana.

Learn more about Dr. Chris at: https://www.nervehealth.com

Other Books by Dr. Chris

The Hidden Diagnosis

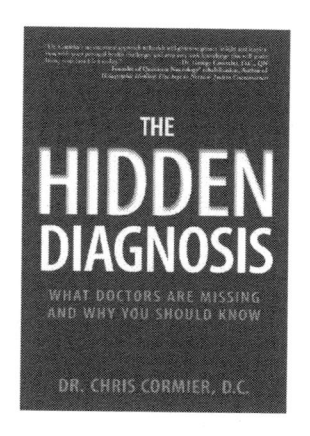

This book uncovers what doctors are missing and explains why you need to know what they're missing. The Hidden Diagnosis is cutting edge and will reveal to you the roadmap to complete health and wellness.

This is a must read for you and anyone you care about. Take a look inside...read the reviews...this book will change your life!

Praise for The Hidden Diagnosis:

Dr. Chris is a true pioneer in neurological thinking! — Dr. Woody Beck, D.C., Q.N.

As a former athlete, I can't believe that I was totally missing this diagnosis in my overall health and athletic performance. This book and these practices are a must for current athletes, former athletes, non-athletes, and everyone in between. — Michael Desormeaux, Former Star ULL Quarterback and Multi-Purpose Player

Dr. Cormier's principles of personal responsibility, whole-body health, and lifestyle shifts ring loud and clear as a playbook for improved wellbeing and health maintenance. — Julian E. Bailes, M.D.

In this book, you will learn:

- Why health is all about your nerves

- How to keep your body running at 100% regardless of your age

- How to fix the root of all disease and sickness

- How to keep your brain connected to all your body's parts

- How to heal the hidden diagnosis lurking inside of you and everyone

God's Amazing Machine

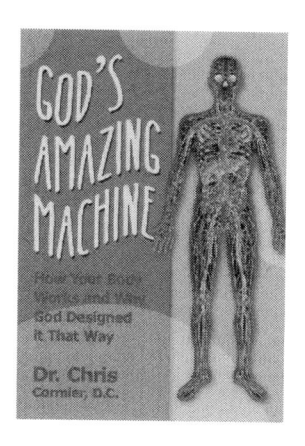

God's Amazing Machine is an enlightening transformational course designed for all types of youth groups nationwide. In seven simple lessons, Dr. Chris Cormier outlines the nature and substance of the human body and the unique value of every person. Guided by a thought-provoking and engaging format, students explore their talents, passions, and purposes, and learn how to honor and maintain their body temples to achieve their greatest potential.

While listening to Pastor Joel Osteen speak on the importance of being thankful, an idea was sparked in Dr. Chris' consciousness. He envisioned a book that would teach children how they could improve their own lives, as well as positively impacting the lives of others, simply by understanding and appreciating what God has already given them—their amazing bodies and the powerful life force that runs through them. This type of education provides a welcome antidote to the raging epidemic of obesity and resulting health challenges that currently threaten our precious young people.

Dr. Chris, who is married to a teacher and has three beautiful children, also had a vision to support teachers by giving them a ready-made, user-friendly system by which to deliver a meaningful curriculum to their students. Well-paced text and a whimsical layout are combined with relevant discussion questions and exercises, designed to stimulate group dialogue and personal connection, giving readers the most enriching experience possible.

Lessons include ...

- Your Body, God, and You Who You Are, A Positive Attitude, What God Wants, How Your Body Works, Disconnection, You Are What You Eat, God's Healing Machine

- God is Love Your Ultimate Creator, Love and Fear, Overcoming Drama, Choosing How You Feel, Knowing How to Pray, God Will Bless You

- God is Light Where is God?, The Light of The World, The Speed of Light, Light is Good for You, Light is Your Source of Power

- The Nervous System — Part I Connection, Communication, Blood Flow, Digestion, Processes

- The Nervous System — Part II Endocrine System, Lymphatic System, Immune System, Muscular System, Respiratory System, Reproductive System

- Interference Choices and Actions, Awareness and Intuition, Intention, The Power of Influence, The Power of Food, Food Labels, God's Guidance, Invisible Interference, Maintaining Your Machine

- Your Will and Determination Desire, Passion, Action, Life Purpose, Being Your Best, Success

Can You Do Me A Favor?

If you enjoyed this book or found it useful, I'd be very grateful if you'd post a short review on Amazon. Your support really does make a difference and I read all the reviews personally so I can get your feedback and make this book even better.

Thanks again for your support!

Dr. Chris

Hyperbaric Oxygen Therapy Burton
Collingwood Ln,
Burton-on-Trent DE13 9SH
Tel: 07857 832969

Printed in Great Britain
by Amazon